PLIABILITY
FOR RUNNERS

THE BREAKTHROUGH METHOD
TO STAY INJURY-FREE, GET
STRONGER, AND RUN FASTER

JOSEPH R. MCCONKEY, MS

USATF Level 3 & World Athletics Level V Coach

Hatherleigh Press is committed to preserving and protecting the natural resources of the earth. Environmentally responsible and sustainable practices are embraced within the company's mission statement.

Visit us at www.hatherleighpress.com and register online for free offers, discounts, special events, and more.

PLIABILITY FOR RUNNERS

Library of Congress Cataloging-in-Publication Data is available upon request.
ISBN 978-1-57826-910-5

All Hatherleigh Press titles are available for bulk purchase, special promotions, and premiums. For information about reselling and special purchase opportunities, please call 1-800-528-2550 and ask for the Special Sales Manager.

Cover and Interior Design by Carolyn Kasper

10 9 8 7 6 5 4 3 2
Printed in the United States

Your health starts here! Workouts, nutrition, motivation, community... everything you need to build a better body from the inside out!

Visit us at www.getfitnow.com for videos, workouts, nutrition, recipes, community tips, and more!

Want to improve your running? The Boston Running Center provides both remote and in-person professional coaching services for runners of all levels. For more information please visit www.bostonrunningcenter.com.

▶ CONTENTS

▶ PLIABILITY:
A GLOBAL CHALLENGE

Addis Ababa, Ethiopia. The air hit the senses before I even got out of the airport, a combination of smells hinting at everything from the tropics to the desert, from farmland to street food. It is the first of many unique experiences one has when visiting the beautiful, vibrant, and resilient country of Ethiopia. Even though this was not my first visit here, this trip became more unique than any other.

I exited the gate and with just a few twists and turns that is the Bole International Airport, I found myself curbside at the passenger pick-up area. Here I waited, hoping my contact Renato Canova, a legendary figure in the world of running, was able to arrange a driver to take me to Sululta, a small village an hour or so outside Addis. I had met Renato during my last trip to East Africa and we had recently agreed to work together for a couple weeks at a High Altitude Training Camp (HATC). As usual, Renato had everything perfectly organized. Immediately, a local Ethiopian man approached me waving with a big smile of familiarity.

"Joe, sir! Welcome back!"

With the bright sun I could not immediately make out who it is, but hearing my name was quite a surprise. Maybe it's a taxi driver, I think; one who just calls all Americans "Joe."

It turned out to be Mersha Asrat: an Addis-based running coach who had attended one of the clinics I had held here two years prior. I was pretty excited to see a familiar face. It seemed like pure luck, and a bit surreal, to enter such a foreign area and have someone recognize me — particularly since it was not planned, and I am not famous.

"Joe, sir," Mersha continues, "I have been learning and practicing every-thing you taught us from last time!"

He actually had a printout in his hand from the clinic, which reminded me how dedicated he was to coaching and learning.

Mersha and I left the airport and caught up on each other's lives over the past couple of years while driving through the city. After an hour or so of weaving through the organized chaos that is Addis rush-hour, Mersha pulls onto the long, dirt road that weaves up into the hills just northwest of Addis, towards Sululta. We soon pass by Haile Gebressalasie's Yaya Village (another HATC), which I look onto fondly, as that was where I had held one of the clinics during my last visit. The landscape is still immac-ulate, the building in great condition, and the little outdoor dining area, amidst meadows, running trails, and forests, is just as it was — a serene place for great conversations amongst diehard (aka crazy) runner people like myself. We cruise on past though, as we are headed to a place I had never seen and only heard about in recent news — the newly completed training camp built by Kenenisa Bekele.

For those who do not follow the competitive and elite faction of running, which I recognize is most of the world, Kenenisa is the undis-puted GOAT. He held the World Record for the 5k and 10k for 16 years (until carbon-fiber plated shoes took over in 2019) and is currently just two seconds shy of the marathon World Record with a 2:01:41 (How heart-wrenching is that!? Two hours of hard running only to miss the world record by two seconds!). He is one of the most famous people in Ethiopia and has a confident but humble personality that draws fans from around the world.

We pulled through the small gate to Kenenisa's HATC, which looks more like a golf resort you might find in Arizona, and stopped just at the entrance to the main building. Mersha got out and walked inside to get logistics organized and I stepped out of the car. I walked onto the immaculate grass lawn, took a deep breath of the crisp, fresh air (much different from the airport), and just about tripped over a runner stretching on the grass.

"Hello," said the man.

I looked down and it was Kenenisa Bekele — right there, right in front of me.

"How's it going?" I casually replied, trying to keep it cool. Renato had mentioned to me that Kenenisa might be around, but I was not expecting to meet him, much less right away. Internally, I was not cool. Thoughts, heartrate, everything was 100 miles an hour.

We engaged in a conversation, with me answering Kenenisa's to-the-point questions like 'Who are you? What are you doing here?' etc. Kenenisa kept saying things like "uh ha' and 'I see' to my responses. He has better things on his mind, I thought.

After a few minutes, Mersha returned. He and Kenenisa spoke Amharic to each other, while I stood there feeling a bit awkward, and then Mersha turned and informed me, "You will work with Kenenisa tomorrow."

Say that again?! I thought to myself, now at 150 mph.

Renato and I had already worked out a schedule for me to work with a specific group of athletes he was coaching at the time, including the entire Chinese Olympic distance team. I could tell, however, that this was not a question from Mersha to me; it was just a statement of fact in terms of what will be occurring. This was confirmed when I looked back to Kenenisa who simply said "See you tomorrow."

First, some backstory: unfortunately, Kenenisa at this point had been suffering perpetual injuries for over five years. The most recent, in his Achilles, was quite severe and had kept him from competition for nearly a year straight. Upon hearing what I focus on, which is basically helping runners create an injury-resistant body, he simply wanted to know more about what it is that I do.

The next day, after meeting with and coordinating logistics with Renato (who was 100 percent behind this change of plans), I was taken back to the city to Kenenisa's hotel and into the hotel gym — which was empty save for Kenenisa and Mersha. I then proceeded to work with Kenenisa on pretty much everything that is discussed in this book.

I first had him stand in front of a mirror and I immediately notice some pretty clear distortions in his standing posture. He is excitingly frustrated, "I have noticed that too but nobody else sees it or mentions it to me."

I found other critical imbalances in his bio-mechanics when running on the treadmill. I took a video and show him. Finally, I had him do a series of stretches and after doing a simple knee-to-chest stretch he said he feels pain in the left hip. I took 1–2 minutes to show him the Targeted Self-Massage idea described in this book, a basic self-massage approach to help relax a muscle and increase circulation. He then repeated the stretch.

"Any difference? Is that better?" I asked.

"Yes, that is better."

He continued, though, to hold the stretch for a bit longer. He seemed to be thinking (feeling?) to himself, fully concentrating on the feedback his body is giving him — a type of 'communication' that elite athletes tend to perfect.

He then looked over to Mersha and says quietly, "Actually, there is no pain at all, it is like…a miracle."

I was immediately apprehensive of that word. I was glad Kenenisa was getting clear feedback from a simple self-care modality, but I quickly mentioned that just because the sensation of pain is gone does not mean the muscle is back to full health. With daily work, however, many of these 'miracle' moments can add up in order to return his body to healthy running. He understood and was excited about the path forward: improve your symmetry of pliability to improve your standing posture to then improve your running bio-mechanics to reduce the asymmetrical load on your legs that has been contributing to the injuries.

After this session, Kenenisa 'claimed' me for the duration of my stay. I discussed this with Renato and he was supportive of the collaboration. It turned out Renato had just started to coach Kenenisa for the marathon but was not making much headway given the injuries. I proceeded to work with Kenenisa for 3–4 hours each day over the next couple weeks. The hours and days flew by. Not only did we get a lot of work done to build his body back to health, but we also got along really well. I met his wife and kids and we had several meals together, at home and out. His celebrity status was visible every time we were in public, with all heads turning and constant requests for autographs and pictures. After a productive and engaging two weeks I wrote out a 'path forward' program for Kenenisa and sat down with him and Mersha, who at the time was just starting to take on the role as Kenenisa's personal running coach. They were very appreciative, with Kenenisa saying, "I wish we had met 5 years ago." I did too.

Soon after my time there, Kenenisa's support team was taken over, first by the Sub2hour initiative started by Dr. Yannis Pitziladis, and then eventually by his agent Jos Hermens and his Global Sports Communication outfit. I was no longer in the thick of the day to day and could only hope my message and approach had stuck with Kenenisa.

Over the next year Kenenisa was able to resume competing. From the video coverage of his races I started to notice subtle improvements in his mechanics. Then, during the 2019 Berlin Marathon, I was happy to notice his form was nearly flawless — level shoulders, no asymmetrical hip rotations, no body lean to the right — and the result…2:01:41. This comes out to 4:39 mile for 26.2 miles — which is just crazy fast!

While Kenenisa is the elite of elite, his predicament was very similar to what I had seen many times before, across all levels of runners, from all corners of the world. It is an injury cycle most runners can identify with. It is also an injury cycle that in most cases can easily be prevented or stopped, on your own, with only 10 minutes per day of your focused attention. The secret?

Pliability.

▶ STOPPING THE INJURY CYCLE

You, too, share certain key physiological traits with elite runners. Are these the same traits that take a person all the way to the Olympics? Perhaps...but for now, we are talking about the all-too-common injury cycle of runners.

Here's how it typically goes for many of us:

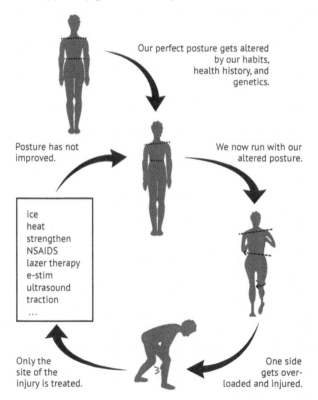

Our perfect posture gets altered by our habits, health history, and genetics.

Posture has not improved.

We now run with our altered posture.

ice
heat
strengthen
NSAIDS
lazer therapy
e-stim
ultrasound
traction
...

Only the site of the injury is treated.

One side gets over-loaded and injured.

Pliability for Runners provides a simple approach to safely stop this cycle. To understand how, let's first address each of the above steps in a bit more detail.

GOOD POSTURE

SYMMETRY

From an injury-prevention point of view, and in my view after working with thousands of runners over the past 18 years, the most important aspect of durable mechanics is symmetry. If the shoulders line over the hips and the hips are level, there is a good chance the legs lift through the area with the same angles, land at the same place on the foot, and have the upper body glide over the hip symmetrically. With this balanced posture you are significantly less likely to develop an injury.

NEUROLOGY

In addition to having more symmetrical movements, a balanced posture also allows for a balanced neurological response. In other words, when your right leg feels tired so does your left, when your right leg feels coordinated and responsive so does your left. It is as if each leg has the exact same radio tower tuned into the same channel. No static, no cross signals.

With symmetrical posture your sensory feedback is more clear, which then allows for smarter decisions — like when to take a rest day, when to slow the pace down, or when to grab the foam roller.

KINETICS

From a performance point of view, symmetry of mechanics also allows for maximum ground reaction forces, aka GRF. GRF is the amount of force from the ground into the body (when you are standing the GRF is simply your body weight, but when you start moving GRF increases due to the acceleration forces into the ground). Let's say your body leans over the right leg more than the left when running.

The GRF into the right leg is going to be very different than the GRF into the left leg. The direction of force will be asymmetrical, the firing of muscles will be asymmetrical, and more than likely parameters like

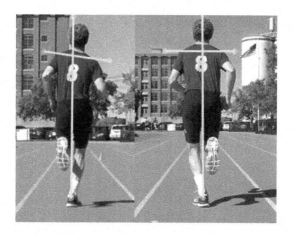

flight time and step length will also be asymmetrical. You are essentially running with one full tire, and one slightly deflated tire.

If your mechanics are balanced, however, you have identical tires that are turning at the same rate, wearing in the same places, and supporting an equal amount of weight. Even if these tires are 'weak', as long as they are symmetrically weak they can now more easily be 'upgraded' (strengthened) through training. In fact, in a recent comparative study it was found that the best 'tires' in the world, i.e. the fastest runners, happen to also be the most symmetrical — the Jamaicans!

REALITY

Do you have to be symmetrical to succeed? Absolutely not. In fact, most people, including elite runners, have some asymmetry. If it is correctable though, or can at least be improved, the chances of staying injury-free, and of building a higher level of power and speed, are greatly increased.

ALTERED POSTURE

POWER OF HABITS

Everything we do, or do not do, can influence our posture. How we stand, walk and run is a product of not only our genetics and injury history, but also of ALL of our habits. Some common contributors to postural distortions are listed in the following 'flow' chart, with the resulting soft-tissue tensions and altered posture.

DAILY HABIT	COMMON TENSIONS	RESULTING POSTURE

SINGLE-SIDE INJURY

Of the runners who have participated in BRC's Gait Analysis Lab over the past 12 years, 90 percent had a history of unilateral injuries, injuries that occur on one leg at a time. In fact, over the last 40 years there have been 14 large studies (500–12,000 participants) on running-specific injuries and with each of these the same 80–90 percent rate of single-side injuries is found. In some rare cases, mostly with beginners, there is a history of simultaneous right and left hip, knee, or shin pain, but for the more regular runners their aches and pains are almost always unilateral.

The runners who have a recurring single-side injury are also just as likely (90 percent) to have a clear asymmetry in their bio-mechanics. One leg rotates outwards, one hip is lower, the body leans one direction more than the other, etc. In other words, there is almost always a clear, logical pathology—a direct connection from how they stand, walk, and run to where their injury is occurring. Though finding the exact cause of every postural distortion is likely impossible, critical cause-effect connections are often too obvious to ignore.

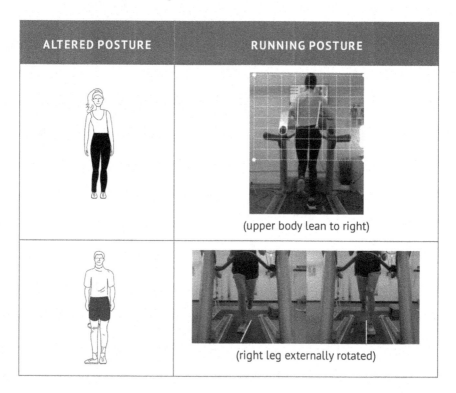

ALTERED POSTURE	RUNNING POSTURE
	(upper body lean to right)
	(right leg externally rotated)

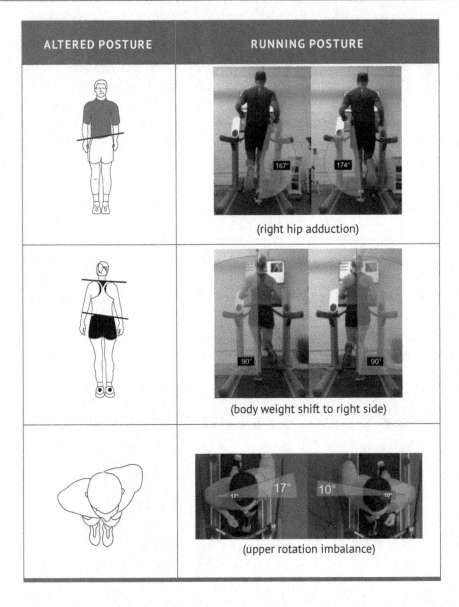

ALTERED POSTURE	RUNNING POSTURE
	(right hip adduction)
	(body weight shift to right side)
	(upper rotation imbalance)

With any of these scenarios the neural feedback is no longer a single clear message. In fact, there is likely opposite sensations coming from each leg. One leg feels like a taught and strong spring, while the other feels like it is made up of Lego pieces that just do not fit together. Each leg is playing its own tune and eventually the 'confusion' will be too much.

RUNNING POSTURE	COMMON INJURY SITE

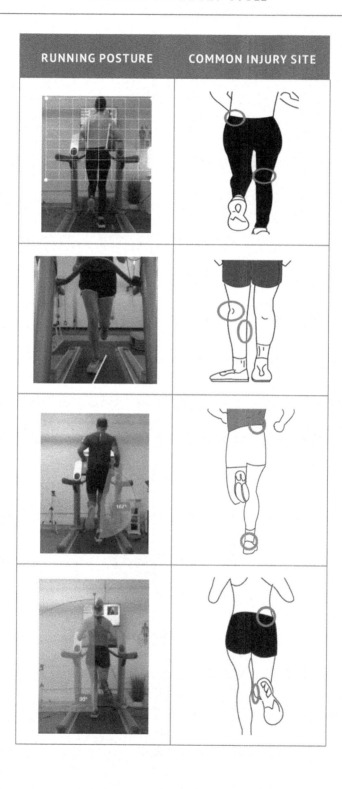

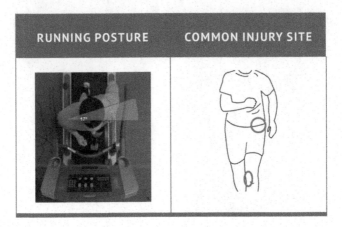

RUNNING POSTURE	COMMON INJURY SITE

In review, a leading contributor for 'over-use' running injuries is an asymmetrical habit or genetic/historical postural imbalance that has worked through and adjusted the posture of the entire body. This altered posture is then put through the act of running and now stresses one side more than the other. Eventually the over-load accumulates into a unilateral repetitive motion injury.

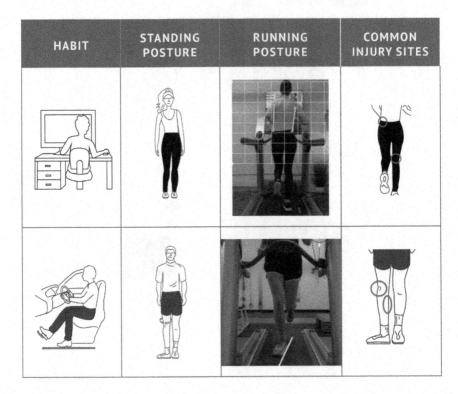

HABIT	STANDING POSTURE	RUNNING POSTURE	COMMON INJURY SITES

HABIT	STANDING POSTURE	RUNNING POSTURE	COMMON INJURY SITES

WHAT EXACTLY IS A REPETITIVE MOTION INJURY (RMI)?

Most injuries for runners come about after an accumulation of many hundreds and thousands of steps, i.e. repetitive motion. With repetitive motion injuries the overload typically starts with very subtle signals. If these signals are not addressed, and the repetitive motion continues, the overload will likely progress into an injury.

WITH AN RMI, WHAT EXACTLY HAPPENS WITHIN THE BODY?

With repetitive motion injuries, the fluid and chemical content within the cells and tissues are altered, including changes in blood pressure, intra-muscular oxidation, and a host of inflammatory and anti-inflammatory agents. This altered chemistry then interacts with soft-tissue, often causing tissue dehydration, microtears, and a hyper-acidic environment.

WHAT DOES AN RMI FEEL LIKE?

With a repetitive motion injury, the muscle is often less compliant to movement, less coordinated, and weaker. The area is typically painful to press, is restricted in mobility, is resistant to compression, and frequently becomes tighter and more painful with more repetitive motion. Here are some common running repetitive motion injuries:

Iliotibial tract syndrome (ITBS)

Achilles' tendonitis

Patellofemoral syndrome

Shin splints

Plantar fasciitis

Piriformis syndrome

Bursitis

Hamstring strain

Calf strain

TREATING ONLY THE EFFECT OF THE INJURY

Injured runners often stop running, think time and rest will fix the problem, and/or they simply provide or get treatment on the specific area of pain. Rarely is the root cause of the injury, which is creating a bio-mechanical imbalance, given full attention. We still wear the phone only on our right arm, sleep on one side of the body, use the mouse with our right hand, run on the same side of a cambered road, rotate our upper body clockwise more than counter-clockwise, our right hip is still higher than the left, on and on. It can become quite clear that our entire body has contorted to a habit and that this is contributing directly to our injuries, yet we still try to 'piece-mail' the solution instead of looking at the issue from a more full-body holistic perspective. Unfortunately, the result of this 'fix what hurts' approach is often a temporary relief, followed by a recurrence of the injury and/or a compensatory injury in a different place of the body.

STOP THE CYCLE!

Iten, Kenya. During another East Africa trip, I was on the Kamariny track, famous because of the world class runners who train there and not because of the actual track, which has a dirt and clay surface with holes and ruts throughout, no lanes, no guard rail, just a 400 meter oval on an empty patch of earth. I was working with Florence Kipligat, who was running out on the roads doing her 3 mile warm up run. On the track were about 50–60 other runners, mostly runners from smaller villages in the Rift Valley. They came to Iten with the hope of training with one of their famous countrymen that they saw on TV winning a marathon or Olympic medal. In other words, they came to Iten with a dream where running was their golden ticket, and they worked very hard to get it.

I learned that twice per week this group would run high volume and very fast workouts on the track, behemoth sessions like 25–30 repetitions of 400 meters at 4 minutes per mile pace, or 20 repetitions of 1 kilometer at a 4:20–4:30 per mile pace. Big workouts, fast workouts (even at altitude), twice per week, on the track, every week. Certainly, these workouts are very challenging, but some runners in Iten are so fit they can absorb this type of schedule, adapt to it, and excel in the sport of running. But I soon found out that for most runners in this group injuries happened all too often. Was there a bio-mechanical reason to this high injury-rate, I wondered? In a matter of hours I found my answer.

Later on that day I came across the same group running their second run of the day, 8 kilometers easy on the roads. As they were approaching my direction, I noticed something off with all of their postures — they were leaning to their left! The road was perfectly flat, with no camber, yet with each of them their left shoulder was much lower, their torso was tilted to the left, and they were all putting more body weight over the left leg while the right hip was taking on a sharper angle of force. It was like they were all still running on the track, where a left-hand curve takes up 50 percent of their workouts. All of those repetitions with high forces put into the left-hand turns seemed to have contorted their body such they their musculoskeletal system was wanting to perpetually turn them left! Immediately I talked with their coach and soon found myself putting the pieces together.

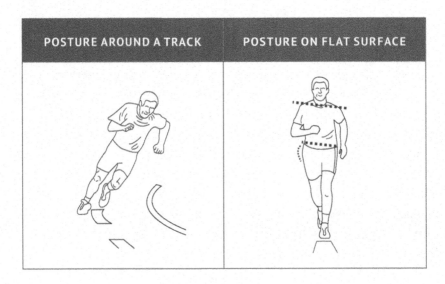

| POSTURE AROUND A TRACK | POSTURE ON FLAT SURFACE |

When working with these 'leaning' runners over the course of the next week (and when working with similar track aficionados throughout the world) I began by having them on a foam roller. Slowly they would roll up, down, right, left all over their legs and back. It was a firework show of grimaces, gasps, and laughs. Sharp pain in left quadriceps, dull ache in the right lateral hip, groaning discomfort from the right lower back. It was quite clear their habits had taken away their natural muscular freedom and the result was now chronic asymmetrical hypertension.

How to stop this cycle? Correct the habit that caused the imbalance? Despite my best efforts, I did not convince the coaches in Iten to have their runners alternate directions on the track. Sometimes tradition is tradition, for better or worse. In fact, in many cases the underlying habit of postural distortions simply cannot be corrected; you still need to drive with your right leg, you have to run on the left side of the cambered road to be safe, you still like to play tennis, etc. When we can't correct the root cause, we're left with the next link in the cycle, which is the resulting asymmetrical hypertension.

If we want to continue an activity where our full body weight is on one leg at a time, such as running, each leg must still be healthy and responding well despite what postural imbalances remain. Does this mean the legs must be equally strong? Perhaps not. For example, folks with scoliosis may have one leg stronger than the other because of a lifetime of an unbalanced weight placed on their hips and legs. Even in these cases, however, each leg must and can be symmetrically healthy. How do you check on the health of your muscles? Pliability.

▶ WHAT IS PLIABILITY?

"I love and believe in pliability. In fact, improving my pliability was a major reason I was able to set the world record while staying healthy and injury-free. Pliability works!"

> —Becca Pizzi, first American to run seven marathons on seven continents in seven days

'P liable' is defined as a person or thing that easily bends or is influenced. It can describe anything from leather, plastic, or wood to the nature of public opinion, and everything in between. In the realm of exercise physiology, the word 'pliability' takes on a similar connotation and can be defined as the ability of our soft-tissue (muscles, tendons, ligaments, fascia) to be compressed without excessive resistance or discomfort. It is a clear, easily deduced physical attribute that many exercise professionals now rely on when assessing an athlete's or client's health and fitness.

"Pliability is the foundation of muscle health. A muscle that is not pliable cannot contract, cannot gain strength or power, lacks nutrition and hydration, is prone to injury and cannot perform as intended."

> —Physical therapist William Hernandez with Delos Therapy

Delos Therapy is a thriving physical therapy practice based out of Chicago and is part of a recent movement in the health/fitness industry. This movement values improving pliability before anything else — before strength, before flexibility, before training. This simple concept has been known and practiced by individuals for decades, and over the past 10 years is moving quickly into the mainstream (including Tom Brady's TB12 training center, where the pliability of NFL football players is valued just as much as pure strength).

As Mr. Hernandez suggested, pliability is perhaps the single most important building block from which a healthy, strong, and coordinated athlete can be fully developed.

ARE YOUR MUSCLES PLIABLE?

If you are pliable your muscles are soft when relaxed, and while relaxed, feel little to no pain if direct pressure is applied. In other words, positions on the foam roll, acute pressure into the muscles of the back, targeted strong thumb pressure into the calf, are all no problem.

If a muscle lacks pliability there is some discomfort and noticeable tension when pressure is applied. A pliable muscle feels like soft Play-Doh, easily absorbing pressure, whereas a non-pliable muscle feels a bit stiff and slightly aches with compression. Here is a side-by-side comparison of a perfectly healthy and pliable muscle versus a chronically hypertensive inflamed non-pliable muscle.

	PLIABLE MUSCLE	NON-PLIABLE MUSCLE
WHAT'S INSIDE	A healthy, stable balance of blood, water, flexible cell walls, responsive protein filaments, and balanced acidity levels.	Thickening of cell walls, strayed muscle fibers, lack of hydration, increased acidity.
WHAT IT FEELS LIKE WITH COMPRESSION	Easy, no pain, no tension, like soft Play-Doh easily wrapping around the pressure of your thumb.	Resistant. The muscle immediately feels tight, not relaxed. Some minor feelings of pain/ discomfort.
REACTION TO EXERCISE	Able to recover quickly and return to a relaxed state. Feels stronger with repeated exercise.	Feels tighter, less pliable after exercise. Maximum strength quickly plateaus.

WHY DOES A LACK OF PLIABILITY AFFECT PERFORMANCE?

When a muscle lacks pliability, that area of the body is likely in the midst of an inflammatory response. This means pro-inflammatory proteins, called cytokines (with 'chicken scratch' names like IL-1β, IL-6, and TNF-α), have flooded the area to localize and reduce damage. This causes an increased sensitivity to pressure, stretching, and perhaps even muscle contraction. Unfortunately, not all damage is repaired by the inflammation response, and not all of the pro-inflammatory agents clear out when their work is done. This leaves an altered chemical makeup within the blood and tissue cells, which then inhibits normal functioning throughout the system. The result is decreased coordination, inhibited super-compensation, and attenuated strength gains.

Why is this so? Envision a desk at a high school chemistry class, covered with tiny vials of various fluids. In this experiment, all of these vials need to be added and subtracted from each other at a specific nano-second or your desk catches on fire! This is how our neuromuscular system works…with perhaps slightly less drama. It is a perfectly executed chemistry experiment, where the passing of positive and negative ions, sodium and potassium exchanges, the opening and closing of synapses within the blood plasma membranes, and the traveling of neighboring neurons within the peripheral nervous system all happen in perfect synchronization.

When a tissue is chronically inflamed, however, the experiment has gone awry. Too much from this vial, not enough from that vial, what's this new vial! In this environment, myogenesis (to repair and build muscle tissue) is no longer possible. The muscle is easily fatigued from exercise, atrophies, and is much more likely to get injured. Not quite the recipe for a PR performance.

For this reason, it is critical to have a healthy, fully circulated, loose and pliable body *before* training. If you don't, and you continually train when your muscles are inflamed, it is like trying to mortar a brick wall together with dry cement. It might stand for a bit but with a slight wind, watch out below!

PUTTING THINGS IN THE RIGHT ORDER

It is unfortunately very common for runners to find out they have a weakness and then immediately start doing strength exercises. A muscle simply will not be as responsive, meaning it will not get as strong as it could, if you are 'strengthening' it when it is tight, stiff, not-pliable. Too help right the wrongs of this relatively small but important part of your world, let's start by putting things in the right order, with pliability BEFORE strength.

PLIABILITY FOR RUNNERS: ORDER OF OPERATIONS

Pliability must be a runner's first priority, before running faster or further and before strength training. But why is this so?

A quick analogy might help us here. Imagine two deflated balloons, each the same exact size. Let's call these our "pliable balloon" and our "stiff balloon." The pliable balloon is full of nothing—just the air that fills the folds of the balloon; the stiff balloon, on the other hand, has a spoonful of sand inside.

Now inflate the two balloons. The stiff balloon with sand inflates quicker, since there was less air space to fill; however, as you continue to inflate, you notice the pliable balloon eventually lifts higher. This is essentially the difference between strengthening a muscle that is pliable versus not pliable. If you strengthen (or run) on a "not pliable" muscle it often reacts like a balloon with sand in it. It contracts (or inflates) quicker but fatigues earlier. This is due to inflammation (sand) and the resulting muscle stiffness, which inhibits circulation, metabolic function, coordination and power.

Okay, we have defined what muscle pliability is, and identified that the benefits of improving pliability extend to injury-prevention, strength training, and your bio-mechanics. Many coaches, athletes, and health practitioners recognize it is a critical piece to optimal performance, and slowly but surely the science community is coming along.

THE SCIENCE BEHIND PLIABILITY

After all the research, and after all the time and money chasing self-claimed miracle cures, most runners will find the most effective and time-efficient way to improve muscle pliability is not by robotic entrapments, vibrating foam rollers, or 'skin burning' creams. Instead, it is through a simple process that has been around for thousands of years — compressive therapy, i.e. massage, done well. Unfortunately, the word massage tends to get a bad rap. Perhaps it is too simple? Takes too much time? Costs too much? Whatever the reason may be, the reality remains that massage is the most time-tested and safest modality to address the majority of the soft-tissue issues that endurance runners come across. So, where is the science to back this up?

Unfortunately, there has been a divide between the medical science industry and the practice of massage for quite some time. Some historians and ethnologists interested in massage even claim this divide stems from the time of ancient Greece, where advances in pharmacology and medical technology were too popular and profitable to ignore, thus pushing out the simple, ancient, and relatively cheap practice of massage. Modern society may have a similar priority, unfortunately, as there is clearly a lack of scientific studies related to massage and its efficacy. Is it from limited finances, resources, or interest? Whatever the reason may be, there are still some noteworthy scientific findings on the topic.

CRITICAL FINDINGS

There have been enough similarly organized studies to unanimously prove that through appropriate 'compression therapy' one can improve tissue compliancy (pliability) to a heightened and lasting level. This more functional state of pliability, these studies show, is the result of several biochemical, biomechanical, and neural reactions, including decreased blood pressure, regained tissue extensibility, and reduced pain sensitivity to pressure.

In addition to these broad, and somewhat subjective findings, some researchers have looked closer, down to the cellular level. The work of Dr. Christin Waters-Baker, and her colleagues at the University of Kentucky, is a leading example. Their studies suggest that macrophages, a key cellular stimulant during repetitive motion inflammation, can be altered from a pro-inflammatory state (M1) to an anti-inflammatory state (M2) through alterations in pressure. Wow! Let's get this straight. In other words, the actual chemical make-up with-in the cells themselves can be changed through simple treatments like massage or foam rolling?! According to the results of Dr. Waters-Baker's work, yes, and the proof is building. In fact, this concept of transferring physical energy (pressure) to chemical energy (altered chemistry) is termed mechano-transduction, and is a process being studied by biochemists and mechano-biologists throughout the world — with exciting findings for the exercise science field hopefully soon to come.

Though the scientific studies involved in massage are limited, they are slowly building each year. Some recent studies even suggest that massage can work better than ibuprofen and may even prevent the growth of cancer tumors! Though much remains to be learned and clarified in the labs, what we can safely retain from past studies is that with appropriate applications of compression, the state of muscle tension and relaxation changes. So what is appropriate? How is massage applied correctly? Unfortunately, on this topic the studies have a clear lack of consistently defined and measured parameters. For example, in most studies the researchers have not measured the exact amount of force to be applied during the compression/massage treatment, or the exact direction and duration of that force. Without this type of consistency and benchmarks, we are a bit stranded by the scientific community and must now turn to empirical evidence for answers. It is here, in this blend of art and science, that *Pliability for Runners* lives.

What follows in these next chapters is a detailed instruction on how to improve your pliability by yourself. It stems from a combination of what has been learned via the scientific method along with what has been learned by athletic coaches, therapists, physiologists, trainers, and runners throughout the world. It is not, however, the 'end all, be all'. Improving your pliability is not going to get you to the Olympics (though it certainly will not hurt your chances). It is also not always the appropriate path for certain people in certain situations. For those wanting a magic pill to heal all their aches and pains, let's first make sure your expectations are appropriate.

Pliability for Runners is an effort to help runners get stronger, faster, and to PREVENT injuries, not cure them. It is an instructional book on how runners can create safe, effective habits in order to help prevent injuries, increase strength, and as a result improve performance. If you are currently injured, this book may not be the best fit for you. In this case, medical care is highly recommended. Physical therapists, physiologists, and running-specific chiropractors and clinical massage therapists, are loaded with education and experience that will make your journey back to health much easier and faster than if you are simply leaving it up to your own findings, intuition, or this book. To get on the same page, let's look more specifically at the progression of running injuries to see exactly where *Pliability for Runners* fits in.

STRAINS VS. SPRAINS

By improving our pliability we are increasing our chances of avoiding common strains. These are distinct from sprains, which are injuries to the soft tissue that connects bones to bones, i.e. ligaments. So here we have our ACL/MCL tears, sprained ankle, or wrist. Sprains are typically brought on by a sudden, acute force or single mis-step. Strains, however, are injuries to soft-tissue that connects muscle to bone, so tendons or a muscle itself. Here we find such gems as hip/glute/quad/hamstring/calf strain, ITBS (you know who you are!), or Achilles tendonitis. Strains can occur from a sudden force/movement, like sprains, but a primary goal of this book is to help runners prevent the types of strains that come about more subtly, through repetitive motion.

FIXING AN ISSUE *BEFORE* IT'S AN ISSUE

A repetitive motion injury (RMI), sometimes referred to as repetitive strain injury (RSI), typically comes about very gradually, with very slight symptoms to start but continually building symptoms if left unattended to. The skills in this book are meant to be learned and applied BEFORE any symptoms, or at the very least, at the absolute earliest sign that something might be off. Let's take a look at the genesis of an injury in a runner, Adam, to understand the typical progression of an RMI and how *Pliability for Runners* might fit in.

ADAM'S CALF INJURY

Adam goes out for an easy run, and towards the last mile of his 4 mile run he notices a slight sensation in his right calf. It lasts for just a few seconds, then goes away. We can call this the 'pre-injury stage'.

PRE-INJURY STAGE

Description: There is no real diagnosis at this stage. It is not a strain, or any sort of label that your doctor could assign to it. Adam just feels that his right calf is slightly 'off' during certain movements or stretches.

Symptoms: Adam feels very slight tension or lack of coordination occasionally while running. When he presses into the calf with his thumb he feels about a 2–3 out of 10. Nothing major, but slightly more than when pressing into the other calf.

Functionality: No issue with regular life. Adam can even run easy and not really feel anything for 90 percent of the run, and the other 10 percent is fine, just something is drawing his attention.

Right here. This is where *Pliability for Runners* fits in — before an injury; or, at the latest, at the 'pre-injury stage'. If you have a very minor sensation that gives off the impression of an upcoming injury, *Pliability for Runners* can fit in perfectly. Anything more than a minor sensation, however, and a medical diagnosis is a must.

Let's go back to Adam and his pre-injury stage. Here is what Adam can hope for:

POST-*PLIABILITY FOR RUNNERS* STAGE

Description: There was some clear imbalances in pliability with several of the self-tests, but now after just a couple weeks of daily TSM (an approach to self-massage described in the next chapter) Adam can no longer feel a difference when pressing strongly into the calf.

Symptoms: Given Adam addressed this issue before it became an injury, he now does not feel the calf at all while running. The calf feels very loose when pressing into it and similar to the other calf. Stretching also feels equal right versus left.

Functionality: Running, walking, stairs are all no problem. Adam can walk on his toes, then on his heels and still no problem. He does notice there is still a weakness in the right calf with one of the self-tests but he is now able to address this through strengthening, given the pliability is now symmetrical.

But perhaps Adam is swamped at work, with two kids bouncing all over him when he gets home. He simply cannot find a way to spend time on fixing himself. Instead, he continues to train with his calf sensation gradually increasing to the point where he feels some pain while running. Eventually, even after some rest, some ice, and Advil, the following happens:

REPETITIVE MOTION INJURY STAGE

Description: A full-on calf strain, perhaps with a minor tearing of the muscle or Achilles tendon.

Symptoms: Everything hurts, even walking.

Functionality: Running is not an option as Adam is gingerly trying to walk without causing further damage.

If you are in a situation similar to the RMI stage, put this book down and call your doctor. *Pliability for Runners* is on the 'pre-hab' side of things, not re-hab!

THE OUTLIERS

Many of the concepts presented in *Pliability for Runners* have been substantiated through clinical study. Some, though, are yet to be fully explored in the labs. For instance, it has never been scientifically proven that being able to perform the squat twist self-test with symmetry of motion will prevent piriformis syndrome (discomfort near the back of the hip). The one commonality that the self-tests and corrective actions presented in this workbook do share, however, is that they have all been developed after years of working with hundreds of runners. They are 'truths' so much as they have tangibly helped the vast majority of these runners. That does of course leave outliers...

If you think you may be an outlier — that is, you are *not* noticing the gains hoped for and described in this book — there are a few extra steps I would encourage you to do. First, re-look objectively at the quality and attention you have given to implementing the corrective actions. Performing the self-tests well, and diligently practicing the corrective actions, can challenge your patience, attention, and discipline. Take a step back, and ask yourself a few questions: Am I really counting slowly to five and applying 10 full compressions with TSM? Did I really practice this self-test for two minutes EVERY day for two weeks straight? In a few instances, I have seen runners conclude they are an outlier too early, when their self-care methods might simply needed to be more consistent or fine-tuned. If after a moment of self-reflection, you still feel this approach is not working for you, please make the effort to seek in-person assistance. A book, by its nature, can never replace the nuanced approach certain situations require.

TAKEAWAY

The skills learned in this book can be helpful only if you are not injured or at the most feel very minor sensations. These sensations should be so minor that if you were to go to your doctor they would likely just say 'well, stop running', and push you right back out through the door. They don't interfere with your regular life, sleep, or even happiness. These sensations are simply something you noticed while running, but can easily forget about. These minor sensations, however, could become far worse if you do not take action—to the point where all the trips to doctors, the sleepless nights, and the chronic discomforts will soon take over your life. You of course want to avoid this at all costs, save for the $20 spent on this book, so you are now ready to be proactive in building an injury-resistant, strong, and efficient running body. If you are uninjured or in the pre-injury stage described above, *Pliability for Runners* might be just what you need to reach your full potential.

▶ GETTING STARTED:
LEARN ABOUT *YOU*

Before improving your pliability let's first learn more about your body, your posture, and how you move. Is this required? Absolutely not. If you would rather move on and get to the part about improving your pliability, feel free to skip forward to the next chapter. No hurt feelings, no harm done. For the rest of you, learning more about your physicality can help explain why you feel or have noticed certain things — like why the shoulder strap falls off of one shoulder but not the other, why one foot always scrapes the shin of the other leg, or why the heel on your right shoe is more worn. Also, connecting the details of your posture to the various levels of hypertension and pliability in your body (which we will get into soon) can be a critical first step to deducing why you are getting hurt, why you lack coordination or balance, and why your performance is perhaps not where you expect it to be.

STANDING POSTURE

This is the first instructional part of the book, so time to stand up! In fact, stand in front of a full length mirror naked or with minimal, tight clothes on. Line up your feet with a tile, board, or line on the floor to ensure your feet are equidistant from the mirror. Now look at yourself in the mirror, taking note of the following:

- **Shoulders:** Are they equal height? Does one sit further back than the other or is one more internally rotated?

- **Trunk:** Is your torso vertical or is it slightly tilted towards one side? Look at the edge of your torso on the right and left sides to help determine this. If you look down is one side of your chest more forward than the other?

- **Hips:** With your first finger of your right hand palpate your right hip bone. Find the front, bony 'knob' or sharp turn of the bone. This is your ASIS (anterior superior iliac spine). Hold your finger steady on the center of this protrusion. Now do the same with your left side. When both fingers are placed in the same spot on the ASIS look down at your fingers and see if one is further forward than the other. Now look at the mirror, is one higher than the other?

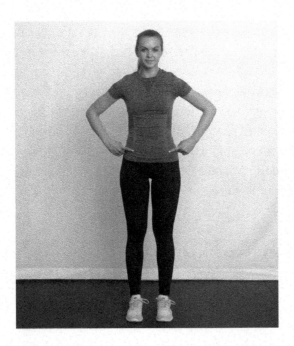

- **Knees:** Look at your kneecaps in the mirror, is one higher? Is one pointed inward? You can also lean over and place your thumbs horizontally above your kneecap, is one thumb higher?

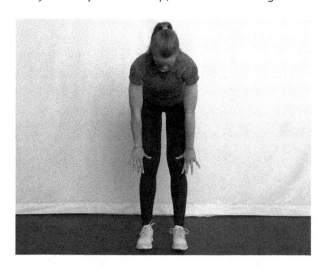

- **Feet:** Look at your feet in the mirror, and by looking down. Does one arch look lower? Is one foot rotated out more than the other?

LYING POSTURE

Lie on your back, arms to the side, barefoot. Make sure you are lying in a straight position. Bring your feet together, do your inner ankle bones meet each other at the same point or do they fit together like a puzzle piece? Perhaps have someone look at your heels to see if they line up. Next, bend your legs, so your feet are flat on the ground. Look up at your knees, are they equal height?

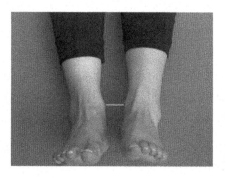
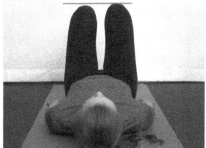

SEATED POSTURE

Seated with legs straight, again look down at the inner protrusion of your ankles (medial malleolus). Are they right next to each other?

Now, place your thumbs in the 'groove' that is just below your kneecap and just above the bony protrusion of your shin bone (the proximal tibial tuberosity). Be sure to relax your quadriceps so that this groove, the patellar tendon, relaxes. Are your thumbs equal distance from you?

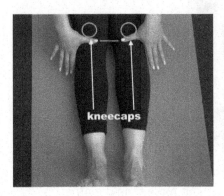 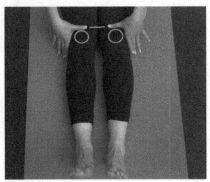

Place your thumbs gently on top of your kneecaps. Are your thumbs equal distance from you?

WALKING POSTURE

While walking naturally, do you notice:

- Is one hand coming further forward than the other or across the body more?
- Does one foot point outward more than the other?
- Does the body rotate one direction more than the other?
- Now take a look at the bottom of one of your most worn pair of walking shoes. Are the shoes worn evenly in the same area?
- If possible, take a video of yourself walking from different angles.
- Does your body lean on one leg more than the other? ("Camera view" from back or front)
- Does one leg cross over your midline of your body more than the other?

RUNNING POSTURE

Repeat the process for walking while running. Here it will become more difficult to self-assess so you may need to seek outside help. Physical therapists or experienced running coaches can help deduce key imbalances or postural distortions in your running gait.

Running imbalances you might be able to notice on your own include:

- One foot pointing outward while on the ground
- One foot swinging outward during the 'swing phase' of your gait
- One foot landing harder or louder
- One hand coming up higher
- Shoulders rotating one direction more than the other
- Different shoe wear pattern on right versus left

Not sure?

Finding postural imbalances may be difficult, and you may be unsure if you are able to notice any differences or the 'correct' differences. Perhaps you are symmetrical, or you are just not used to noticing slight differences in your body. Though minor asymmetries are critical, as discussed earlier, noticing them at this stage is not. Try your best, but if still unsure, move forward trusting your instincts and knowing that the most critical skill of improving your pliability will rely not on your visual analysis, but your sensory feedback.

TO FIX YOUR FORM OR FIX YOUR BODY?

Have you noticed your body is unbalanced when you run? Or that you tend to lean over or backwards too much? Do you notice a difference with how you look when you run vs an elite runner on TV? If so, perhaps you have searched online 'good running form', then grabbed a couple running 'method' books like ChiRunning, Pose Method, etc. and went about the project of improving your form. For those that have, you likely noticed a difference in how you run, and perhaps even avoided injuries and got a bit faster. If so, that's great! But what happens when you strive for your full potential? What happens when you advance your training beyond easy running and higher volume? What happens when you try to run fast *and* far? In my experience this is where the popular running method books fall short — which perhaps explains why elite distance track runners do not practice these methods (elite meaning 800 meter to marathon runners who are running 3:20–5:20/mile pace).

The fact is, to run fast for long distances you need to be able to generate and absorb a lot of force, which takes a high level of strength and dynamic flexibility. It involves not just high-volume training, but also high-quality training. Running with images of circles around your knees, or a stick connecting your heel to your shoulder can help with your general mechanics but will it protect you when you are running through high levels of stress and fatigue? After working with beginner to world-class runners of all shapes and sizes, I am not convinced. Runners who want to run injury-free *and* reach their full potential (run their fastest) are better served by learning how to take care of their body, more than relying on their ability to be in the 'perfect' position all the time, even when running tired. Yes, form matters, and asymmetrical bio-mechanics cause most running injuries, but the safest place to start is the cause of the asymmetry, and in most cases that starts with pliability.

YOUR CURRENT PLIABILITY

Before learning if and what needs to be improved with your current pliability, let's establish a baseline of where things are right now. For this you will need to pick up a foam roller, as this will be the easiest way to apply pressure throughout most of the body. If you don't have a foam roller, look for a 3' long, 6" diameter high density foam roll online or at your local sports/running store:

Next, apply pressure from the foam roll into your body while in various positions. While doing this it might be best to take notes and apply a scale 0–10 for each position for each side. The scale should be defined something like the following:

PLIABILITY ASSESSMENT SCALE

0 No pain, no discomfort, no tension; it feels like the muscle is relaxed and you feel fine, comfortable

1 Almost nothing, perhaps a very slight sensation of tension

2 Some tension/resistance in the muscle to the pressure, but manageable

3 Immediately noticeable tension/resistance to pressure; feels okay but not fully relaxed

4 You feel some tension, almost slight discomfort; a 'good' kind of hurt

5 Definite tension, slight discomfort; it feels like something you should work on, but you are also okay keeping the pressure on for a while

6 There is clear discomfort right away, you can still relax, but the tension is noticeable

7 Tension and discomfort are acute sensations you feel right away, this is no longer becoming fun

8 You immediately want to move the pressure away, it is that uncomfortable, but you can hold it and stay relaxed if you have to

9 The tension and discomfort sensations are very loud; muscle feels tight and not happy

10 Immediate withdrawal; too much discomfort to handle

POSITION 1: GLUTES

Sit on the foam roll and slightly twist your body to the right, so that you feel the pressure of the foam roll directly into your right glute. Slowly move around, rotating 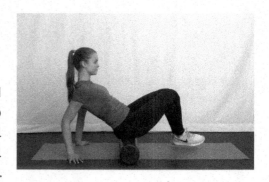 the body clockwise and counterclockwise, sliding right and left lengthwise along the foam roller, and rolling forward and backwards. All movements should be very slow so that you can accurately assess the tension without causing the muscle to tense up as a reaction to the movements. 'Assign' a number, 0–10, to what you are feeling and switch sides.

POSITION 2: QUADRICEPS

Lie facing down, placing your right hip on the foam roll. Slowly roll 3–5 inches down the front of the leg, then back to the hip. Repeat, slowly rolling back and forth. Assign a number 0–10. Next, repeat the slow back and forth roll-ing, now in the middle of the 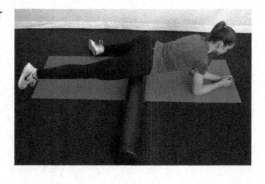 right thigh (quadricep). Assign this area a number 0–10. Finally repeat and assess the area of the quadricep just above the knee, assigning a number 0–10.

POSITION 3: HAMSTRINGS

Place the foam roll on a chair, high table, or counter. Sit on the foam roll such that the foam roll is pressing into the middle of the back of the leg. Cross one leg over the other and lean over so that your upper body is over your legs. Slowly rotate the body, glide right or left, or roll back and forth. Assign 0–10 to the pliability level you are feeling.

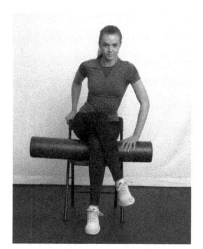

POSITION 4: CALVES

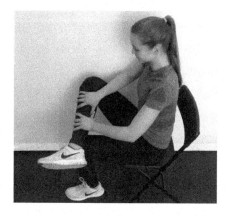

Cross your legs, wrap your fingers around the shin bone, stack your thumbs over each other, and press the thumbs strongly into the center of the calf muscle. You will essentially be compressing the calf muscle between your thumb and the shin bone. Use your fingers to squeeze and provide more pressure. Release and replace the pressure to a nearby area. Continue replacing and assessing the pressure into the calf, assigning a number for the maximum amount of tension felt.

Find any imbalances with your pliability? If so, the time to improve your pliability is now! Failing to address this imbalance while continuing to run is the most common causes to overuse injuries. So without further ado, let's get to the good stuff!

► IMPROVING PLIABILITY IS IN *YOUR* HANDS

To improve pliability, you do not need to hire a massage therapist, physical therapist, or even find a partner. You only need yourself, perhaps a tool or two mentioned later in this chapter…and *10 minutes of your day.*

FREQUENCY

As mentioned earlier, the most effective way to improve pliability is through compression therapies such as a massage, foam roller, lacrosse ball, etc. How often is this needed? To answer this, remember most asymmetrical hypertensions that have occurred from running likely took many thousands of minor 'miss'-steps to get to its current state. With this frequency of a repeated signal, it will take a similar frequency of a 'counter' signal to reverse. So, thousands of massages? No, in fact walking, much less running, would be difficult at that point! What we do need, though, is daily pliability work for at least two weeks. That is every day, seven days per week, with no misses.

SELF-MASSAGE

"Self-massage is one of the most important things you can do to stay injury-free as a runner."

> —Julia Kirtland, former elite runner and licensed massage therapist

43

Given the infeasibility of having a professional massage therapist available every day, runners must develop the skills to provide compression therapy on themselves. For simplicity we'll call this 'self-massage', which includes the use of any tools like a foam roll, Thera Cane, lacrosse ball, etc. Self-massage, for many, is a vague, general idea. The secret 'magic' of it hides in a secret dark cave, where very simple and specific details of its inner workings can be found. It is time to enter that cave, with a big bright flashlight leading the way. Your pliability, which dictates your health and strength, depends on it.

TARGETED SELF-MASSAGE

In terms of making real, lasting changes in pliability there are good and bad ways to provide self-massage. Movements that are too fast, or compressions that are not held long enough, can have minimal or even negative effect on the tension of a muscle. Whereas a held, focused pressure with slow movement can make a world of difference. The following approach is derived from several health and fitness specialists, including other BRC coaches/therapists; Eric Owens, co-founder of Delos Therapy; and myself. This approach is called 'targeted self-massage' (TSM) and serves as the essential skill of *Pliability for Runners*. Read through the detailed instructions carefully. Internalize them, remember them, and be prepared to use your new skill of TSM with the self-tests and corrective actions in later chapters.

TARGETED SELF-MASSAGE

1. **Direct pressure:** Apply strong, static, and focused pressure directly into the tightest part of the muscle and hold for 3–5 seconds. Note this tension should be no more than a 6 on the Pliability Assessment Scale on page 39. If the tension is more than a 6, reduce the pressure or soften the surface—for example, put a blanket on the foam roll, or do the foam rolling on a carpet—so that the tension is in the 0–6 range.

2. **Stretch movement:** During the 3–5 seconds, slightly move the direction of force in one direction only. In other words, while pressing directly into the muscle, next press slightly upwards, or slightly downwards, to the right, left, clockwise, or counterclockwise—which ever direction you feel a slight increase in stretch or tension within the muscle. Note with this movement you are not sliding along the skin, but are simply trying to both compress (direct pressure) and stretch (oblique pressure) the muscle simultaneously.

3. **Release and relax:** After the 3–5 seconds, release all pressure, relax for 1–2 seconds, then re-apply the direct pressure in the same exact area and again hold for 3–5 seconds. Change the direction of the stretch movement if little to no tension was felt with the direction of the last movement.

4. **Repeat 10 times:** Continue to re-apply the direct pressure + stretch movement for 3–5 seconds at a time on the same area of tension for a total of 10 cycles, typically 60–90 seconds per area.

5. **Repeat daily:** Repeat the 10 cycles of sustained pressure one to three times per day.

Let's work through an example of how to apply TSM. For this example we'll focus on the glutes. When in the below position, let's say you feel a 4–5 out of 10 with the pressure into the right glute and only a 0–1 in the left.

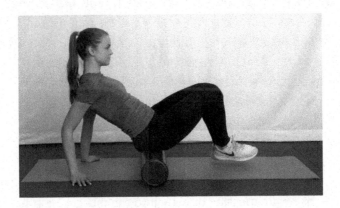

To apply TSM to the right glute, hold steady pressure for 3–5 seconds into the area that feels the tightest, again with no more than a 6 out of 10 tension.

During the 3–5 seconds move slowly in one direction only, not back and forth, all while continuing to hold the pressure in the same exact area. This means you can rotate in one direction, or glide right or left.

DO NOT ROLL!

In order to keep the pressure steady, in the same area, this means with TSM you are never rolling! Rolling would mean you are moving the pressure off and on the area of tension. Instead TSM involves providing focused targeted pressure in a single, specific area of tension. The *stretch movement* of TSM provides a change in the direction of pressure, not where you are applying the pressure.

FILL YOUR TOOLBOX

Though the foam roller is a great tool to help you easily apply strong pressure, sometimes you need more acute pressure to make a real, lasting improvement in pliability. When this is the case your hands and thumbs are always recommended, as the tactile feedback can be instrumental in learning what slight changes in pressure or position are helpful. If you do not have strong enough hands, or the area is hard to reach, like the back of your shoulder, it would be best to add one or two key items to your homecare kit.

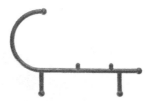

Thera Cane: A green hook with knobs, approx. $25

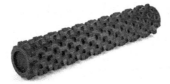

Rumbleroller: 31″ by 6″ diameter, approx. $45 (a bit pricier but well worth it)

Other tools can be helpful, including a lacrosse ball, PVC pipe, even a can of soup! Whatever tool you have, use it well. Apply the TSM approach with the tool, and pay close attention to the details of movement, as you would if you were using your hands.

PLIABILITY AND NUTRITION

A healthy, strong and pliable muscle needs a bit of everything to function at its best — carbohydrates, proteins, fats, vitamins, and minerals. Each serves a critical function in muscle functioning, which are defined, albeit in an over-simplified manner, below:

- Protein: Builds muscle
- Carbohydrate: Provides energy to muscle
- Fats: Helps with recovery and repair of muscle

- Calcium: Initiates muscle-firing
- Vitamin C: Growth and repair of muscle tissue
- Vitamin D: Regulates calcium, assists in growth and repair
- Iron: Provides oxygen to muscle
- Water: Enables everything above to do their jobs

If one or more of these nutrients are deficient in the muscle, that fine-tuned chemistry experiment has again gone awry. So, in short, eat a well-balanced meal and stay hydrated in order to gain and maintain your pliability.

TIME COMMITMENT

A key thing to note about TSM is that it does not take much time. In fact, to notably improve your pliability you typically only need to dedicate 10 minutes each day. For some, however, even finding 10 minutes in their day can be difficult. For those folks, unfortunately, their problems might continue perpetually. If you cannot find 10 minutes in your day, or you simply forget to take care of yourself in-between runs, your body does not forget about your accumulating tensions. The body will not just give you a break and say, 'Well, Right Calf is unhappy and might cause pain for a while, but since you are so busy, I'll fix you up this time while you jump on your conference call.' If only mind and body had such a relationship! Instead, our body reacts to everything we do or do not do, regardless of our busy lives.

So our first goal is to find the time. Find 10 minutes per day dedicated to building a more injury-resistant you. What about runners with a history of running injuries but who are not able to fit in that extra 10 minutes? This is where an activity with less force might be the best option (e.g. swimming, biking, elliptical). If you are committing to 10 minutes per day, though, and your 10 minute habit started by reading this book, let's learn next *where* exactly we should be improving our pliability.

▶ SELF-TESTS:
RANGE OF MOTION

At this point we've learned the basics of pliability — what it means to be pliable, how to assess your own pliability via the foam roller, how to improve your pliability via the TSM approach. The last, and most critical piece, is to know *where* to improve your pliability.

Kristen, 37 years old, ran 40–45 miles per week and on her good years qualified for and ran the Boston Marathon. Recently though, she was getting right knee pain (patellofemoral syndrome) when she would get close to 40 miles per week and was not sure what to do about it. She wanted to run more and get faster but was not able to get the training in due to this 'pre-injury'. She had gone to physical therapy and there they found her right quadricep was tight and weak. Perfect, off she went with regular foam rolling and leg extension exercises and soon her quads felt equally loose and equally strong. She started building up her volume with no problem, but again when she neared the 40 miles per week mark, the knee pain returned and this time it was even worse! She was confused and frustrated, and that is when I met her.

Upon further investigation, her right leg rotated inwards when she ran (likely stemming from a hip obliquity — as one hip was higher than the other when she was standing). Her right glute was significantly tighter than the left on the foam roll, and she could only do 10 glute bridges with her right leg where with her left she could do 20. So that's it! The quadricep was tighter because it was trying to protect the right knee due to the weakness of the right glute. Given the gluteus medius works with the medial quadricep to stabilize the knee, if the right glute is tight and dysfunctional, improving the health and function of the right glute will ease the load on the quadricep, and thus ease the tension into the tendon and greatly reduce the chance of injury. Right? Maybe, but maybe not!

In this case, even further investigation showed she was severally limited in rotating her torso to the left and she felt clear tension in the right lower back when attempting to do so. The fact is the right glute and the right erector spinae of the lower back work together to keep the pelvis in place. So, logic fuels the train further along the tracks — improving the health and function of the right lower back will ease the tension of the right glute, which in turn will ease the tension of the right quadricep and thus the tendon into the knee, and no more injury. But wait! Did the right lower back tension come from her posture at the computer, or is there something else? The investigation is not over and must cover all possibilities!

Fortunately, we were able to trace the right lower back tension to a previous shoulder injury. After 6 weeks of following a comprehensive program to rebuild symmetrical pliability and strength *throughout* her body, Karen was easily absorbing 60+ miles per week. All with 10 minutes per day, focusing on only, and exactly, what mattered.

Kristin's situation exhibits the most common problem I find with the majority of diagnostic protocols, and their recommendations. Too often the interconnectedness of the entire soft-tissue system is not considered and the recommended corrective actions are too specific. Given this, rather than simply poking around and providing TSM to areas that hurt, we need to have a more full-body approach. To do this *Pliability for Runners* uses simple movements of the body, movements that are closely related to the act of running. These movements not only show us where to apply TSM, but they also serve as a test, telling us if the TSM we are providing is actually making a real difference. Here is an outline of how the process works:

RANGE OF MOTION (ROM) SELF-TESTS: HOW THEY WORK

1. Perform the self-test, which will be some sort of single-side stretch or movement. Compare right vs. left flexibility, noting if one side feels tighter than the other.
2. Perform TSM on the area that feels like it is restricting the stretch or movement and is keeping it from feeling symmetrical.
3. Repeat the self-test, noting if there is improvement.
4. Repeat #1–3 for 1–3 cycles every day for 2–4 weeks.

Before working through the self-tests, our last bit of homework is to learn which positions you can safely and effectively apply TSM to various parts of the body. The following suggested positions are not definitive and subtle variations can certainly be helpful, but for now take a glance through and remember to refer back to these pages when working through the self-tests.

TARGETED SELF-MASSAGE (TSM) POSITIONS

1. QUADRICEPS AND HIP FLEXORS

Remember not to roll, but to hold the pressure. If you add a slight movement, it should be one where you are rotating or gliding lengthwise along the foam roll, i.e. where you are slightly pulling the tense area instead of rolling off and on it.

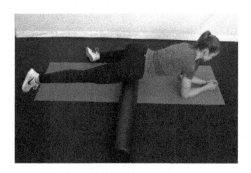

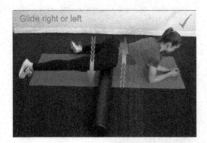

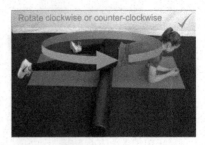

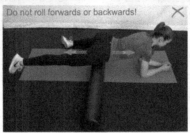

2. HIP FLEXORS

Here you are pressing your thumb into the hip flexor (the top portion of the front of your leg). With the leg bent the hip flexor should be shortened and relaxed, which would allow for higher quality TSM. Place your opposite hand over the thumb to provide more pressure. Note, this position can also be done while standing, with the leg bent and on a chair.

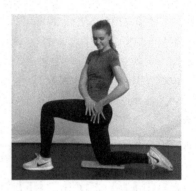

3. QUADRICEPS AND HIP FLEXORS

Again, you are pressing the thumb into the front of the thigh in order to apply TSM. You can also lean over to slacken the hip flexor and/or to address the mid-quadricep area.

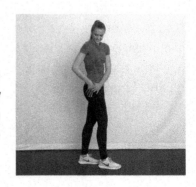

4. GLUTES

To apply TSM, roll the Thera Cane to the side to pull the end into the glute, and/or pull upwards toward the ceiling. Remember to hold the pressure steady with only a single small movement for every 5 second compression.

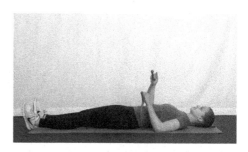

5. GLUTES

Note the hips come forward and the slight backward lean of the trunk, all so the glutes are shortened and slackened. Pull/push the Thera Cane inward, forward to apply TSM. If you have strong hands, thumb pressure might be best in this position.

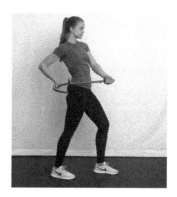

6. GLUTES

Again: hold, do not roll. If any movements are added they should be rotational or lateral gliding movements. Remember to release pressure for 1–2 seconds after 3–5 seconds of compression.

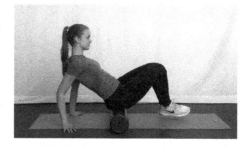

7. LOWER BACK

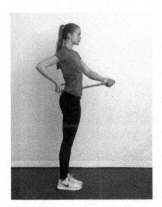
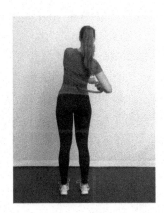

Adjust your position so the area is slackened and loose, perhaps leaning to one side, leaning back, or standing with legs wide, or staggered. Push/pull the Thera Cane (or your thumb) inward and forward to apply TSM.

8. LOWER BACK

Relax and allow the back to 'sink' around the Thera Cane. Try with legs bent and feet on floor, or straight and wide apart. Pull the Thera Cane upwards, towards to the ceiling, to apply TSM.

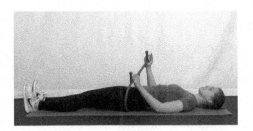

9. UPPER BACK

Press the end of the Thera Cane into the upper back, pressing inward and forward to apply TSM. Slightly pull the Thera Cane right, left, up or down to add the oblique force to the targeted, direct pressure.

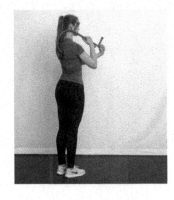

10. HAMSTRINGS

The bottom leg should be relaxed and bent so the hamstring is shortened and slackened. Cross the opposite leg over and lean over so maximum weight is over the leg. Remember, do not roll when applying TSM, the movement should be a rotation or glide. If this is 0–1 out of 10, try this on the rumbleroller! A healthy runner can sit like this on the rumbleroller and still feel 0–1.

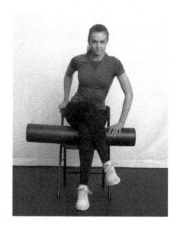

11. HAMSTRINGS

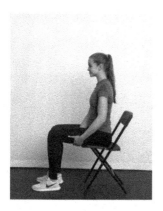
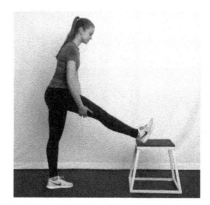

Stack fingers of right and left hand over each other to apply stronger, more targeted self-massage. You can also bend the leg to slacken and loosen the hamstring. Note, with the straight leg position shown you can also address the quadricep.

12. HAMSTRINGS

This position is great for addressing hamstring tension found in the 'lying knee to chest' self-test. Have a chair nearby so you can quickly relax, shorten, and slacken the hamstring.

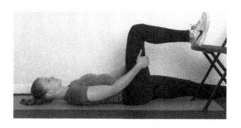

13. CALVES

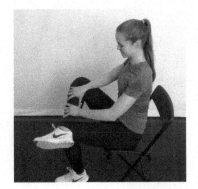
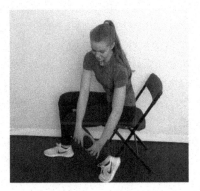

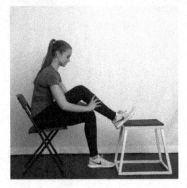

Stack the thumbs over each other so that you can apply strong and targeted pressure, countering the pressure from the fingers against the shin bones. In the first picture, where the foot is free, off the ground, the stretch movement of TSM can be applied by pointing the foot down, and then up, all while holding the pressure constant with your thumbs.

14. SHINS

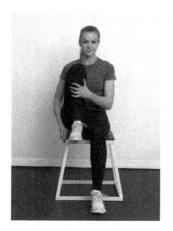 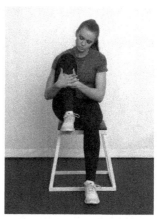

Place the opposite hand over the shin bone, with fingers wide and grappling the shin muscle (left picture). Press your fingers inwards, towards the shin bone to provide TSM. Note, your palm should be on the opposite side of your shin bone, providing additional resistance and strength. Place and press the opposite hand over the fingers to provide additional pressure (right picture). The stretch movement can be applied either by changing the direction of force of your hands, or by lifting the toes up and then slowly pointing them down.

These TSM positions are certainly not exhaustive and should be used only as an initial reference. Feel free to make adjustments so that you feel you are able to easily apply strong, direct pressure to the area of focus.

GENERAL GUIDELINES WHEN FINDING A POSITION TO APPLY TSM:

- Get in a position where the area is loose, i.e. not contracting.
- Get in a position where the area is slackened, i.e. not being stretched.
- Get in a position where you are comfortable. You should easily be able to apply strong pressure if needed. Use tools like the Thera Cane to help with this.

Now that we have an understanding of the TSM positions, let's move forward and walk through the first Range of Motion (ROM) self-test!

#1: **Standing Torso Twist**

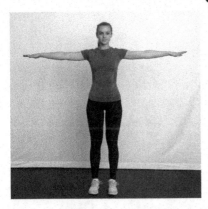 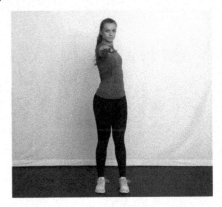

PLIABILITY GOALS

- Symmetry of soft-tissue restrictions
- Symmetry of range of motion

SELF-TEST INSTRUCTIONS

1. Stand with feet hip width apart and arms up, as shown.

2. Slowly rotate your body clockwise as far as you can comfortably go. Arms, trunk, hips... all can move. Hold this position for a few seconds and pay attention to any areas of the body that feel like they are being stretched.

3. Now rotate in the opposite direction, again holding and paying attention to any feelings of tension, restriction, or stretching.

4. Compare if one direction was more restricted, and if you felt a stretch or tension in different areas of the body.

CORRECTIVE ACTIONS

- Provide TSM to asymmetrical areas of tension and re-test.

#1: EXAMPLE AND INSTRUCTIONS

First, stand with feet hip width apart and arms up, as shown.

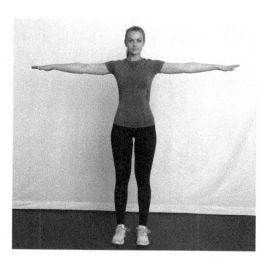

Slowly rotate your body clockwise as far as you can comfortably go—arms, trunk, hips all can move. Hold this position for a few seconds and pay attention to any areas of the body that feel like they are being stretched.

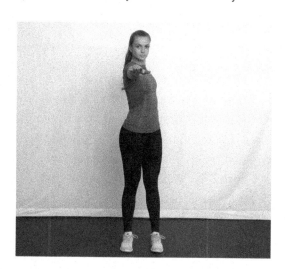

Now rotate in the opposite direction, again holding and paying attention to any feelings of tension, restriction, or stretching.

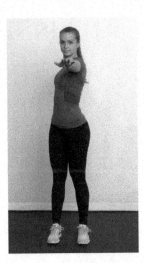

Compare if one direction was more restricted, and if you felt a stretch or tension in different areas of the body. It might be helpful to take notes, so you can track changes later on. A sample chart is below:

DATE	ROM SELF-TEST	LEFT	RIGHT
MM/DD/YYYY	Standing Torso Twist	Felt fine, no real stretch	More restricted, tension in right lower back

On the bottom of each ROM self-tests you will see, 'corrective actions: Provide TSM to asymmetrical areas of tension and repeat test.' This means if specific, asymmetrical soft-tissue restriction was felt, perform TSM on the restricted area. For example, let's say you felt clear tension in the right lower back when trying to rotate clockwise. The next step is to look through the TSM positions on pages 51–57 and to find a position that targets the area you felt was restricting the movement from feeling like the opposite direction/side. In this case, TSM position #7 hits the spot!

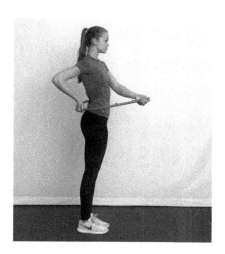

In this position, place the Thera Cane in the area you felt was restricting the torso rotation and apply TSM as described on page 54. This means, apply pressure by gradually pulling the Thera Cane inwards. If there is no tension, move an inch or so to a different, but nearby area and re-apply the pressure. Try all directions of pressure when assessing — directly inwards, inwards and up, inwards and down, inwards and to the left, etc. When you find there is more than a 0 out of 10, compare this tension to the same area on the opposite side. If indeed there is an imbalance, perform TSM.

'Re-test' is the last part of the corrective action. After providing 10 cycles of TSM, re-test the Standing Torso Twist. Slightly better? In most cases you should notice some improvement right away, after just one cycle of self-test-TSM-re-test. Your next job is to repeat this process every day! With daily work many imbalances of this nature will take just 2–4 weeks to improve to a more permanent state of symmetry.

SO, ROM SELF-TESTS, IN SUMMARY, WORK AS FOLLOWS:

1. Perform the stretch, comparing right vs. left
2. Apply TSM to the restricted area
3. Re-test the stretch
4. Repeat #1–3 (self-test/TSM/re-test) every day until symmetrical

After going through the standing torso twist self-test, we now move on to the next self-test with a similar approach. Before doing so, a few more tips and considerations.

TIPS WHEN PERFORMING ROM SELF-TESTS

FOCUS. Select a time and space where you will be left alone, in a quiet area without distractions.

BE PATIENT. As you work to gain range of motion, take note you might be working against chronic tension that has taken years to develop, perhaps after thousands or millions of slightly imbalanced strides. Be patient as you look for signs of minor improvement every few days.

BE CREATIVE. Though it takes time and consistency to make lasting improvements you should feel minor improvements every day, and quickly! If this is not happening, something may need to change. Perhaps a slight change in position, or a slight change in the amount or direction of the compression, for example.

DRINK WATER AND EAT HEALTHY. Much of a lack of pliability and range of motion comes from lack of fluid flow and essential anti-inflammatories and hormones within the cells. If we are trying to mobilize fluid and fluid content, let's make sure we have a built-up reservoir of clean energy to draw from!

MANAGE YOUR TIME. Creating new, efficient daily habits is the most critical step towards becoming more injury-resistant. If you truly only have ten minutes a day to work on improving your imbalances, that is not a problem, you can still expect to improve rapidly. In this case only work on 1–2 tests each day, just 3–5 minutes per test. When you pass a test, continue to retest that movement every day. If the gains you made are holding, each test will soon take just 3–5 *seconds* as you quickly notice there are no longer asymmetrical tensions. When you have reached this point you now have time to move on to the next test. The final goal is to go through all 15 ROM tests in one day in about 3–4 minutes total! In most cases, this can only be achieved with daily work over 1–2 months.

TRUST YOUR INSTINCTS. If you have given enough time, have slowly performed the movement, and you still do not notice any imbalances, you are most likely right. At the very least the imbalance may be too minor to be concerned about with this step. In this case, move on and trust if something important was missed it will present itself more clearly in later tests.

START AND MAINTAIN NEW HABITS. Don't assume if one day you pass a test (e.g. you feel symmetrical range of motion when pulling knee to chest) that you will always be this way. Perhaps you spent a day gardening, or ran a hard hill workout too soon, or sat in an odd position on a plane. All of this can cause soft-tissue tensions to creep in. Start a habit of regular check-ins, more on this to come!

Let's now apply all the lessons covered so far with the remaining ROM self-tests.

#2: **Shoulder Mobility Screen**

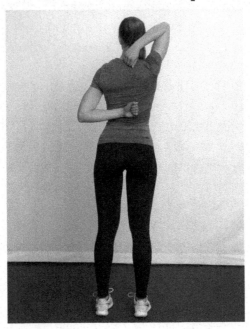

PLIABILITY GOAL

- Symmetry of soft-tissue restrictions

SELF-TEST INSTRUCTIONS

1. Attempt to touch your fists together as shown. Look in a mirror or have someone note how close your fists are.

2. Repeat the test with the opposite set-up.

3. If one fist can reach higher or lower than the other, note if there is an area of specific tension that is restricting the limited side.

Corrective Actions

- Provide TSM to asymmetrical areas of tension and re-test.

#3: **Supermans**

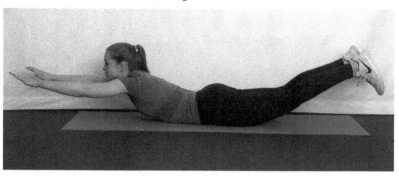

PLIABILITY GOAL
- Symmetry of soft-tissue restrictions

SELF-TEST INSTRUCTIONS
1. Lie on the ground as shown. Lift both arms and legs up as high as possible.
2. Note if any asymmetrical tensions occur (shoulder, back, glutes, hamstrings).

CORRECTIVE ACTIONS
- Provide TSM to asymmetrical areas of tension and re-test.

#4: **Lying Torso Twist**

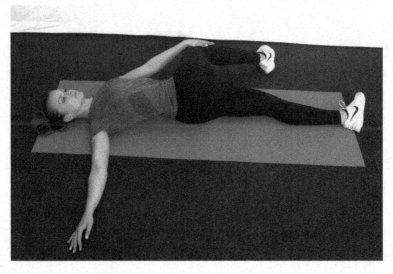

PLIABILITY GOAL
- Symmetry of soft-tissue restrictions

SELF-TEST INSTRUCTIONS
1. Lie on your back.
2. Place your left hand around your right knee, and your right arm out to the side (as shown).
3. Slowly rotate your trunk, lightly pulling your right leg to the ground while keeping your right elbow on the ground.
4. Repeat with the opposite side.

CORRECTIVE ACTIONS
- Provide TSM to asymmetrical areas of tension and re-test.

#5: **Squat Twist**

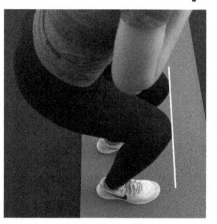 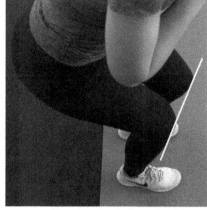

PLIABILITY GOAL
- Symmetry of soft-tissue restrictions

SELF-TEST INSTRUCTIONS
1. Stand with feet hip width apart and lower down to a squat position (thighs just above parallel to ground).
2. While keeping your knees pointing in front of you, pull one leg straight back as much as possible. Avoid rotating your hips and stay in a low squat position throughout. Hold for 3–5 seconds, noting areas of tension, if any.
3. Repeat, now pulling the opposite leg back

CORRECTIVE ACTIONS
- Provide TSM to asymmetrical areas of tension and re-test.

#6: **Knee to Chest**

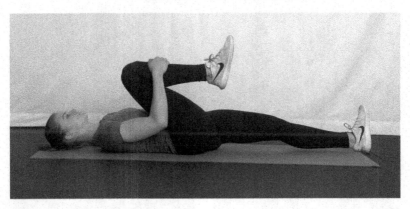

PLIABILITY GOAL
• Symmetry of soft-tissue restrictions

SELF-TEST INSTRUCTIONS

1. While lying on your back, pull one knee down towards your chest (as shown).

2. Note any stretch in the hamstring/glutes, or pinch in the hip.

3. Repeat with the opposite leg.

CORRECTIVE ACTIONS
• Provide TSM to asymmetrical areas of tension and re-test.

#7: **Knee to Chest with Twist**

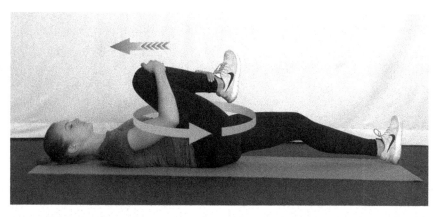

PLIABILITY GOAL
- Symmetry of soft-tissue restrictions

SELF-TEST INSTRUCTIONS
1. While lying on your back hold one leg twisted at around a 45° angle, one hand on the ankle and one around knee.
2. Pull the shin up and across the body, towards the opposite shoulder, with equal pressure from right and left hands.
3. Repeat with the opposite leg.

CORRECTIVE ACTIONS
- Provide TSM to asymmetrical areas of tension and re-test.

#8: **Hip Flexor Active-Isolated Stretch**

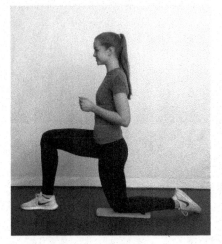
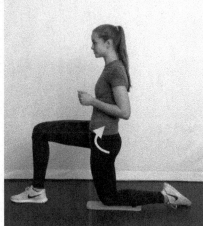

PLIABILITY GOAL
- Symmetry of soft-tissue restrictions

SELF-TEST INSTRUCTIONS
1. Kneel as shown, with the hip of the down leg directly over the knee (do not lean forward).

2. Contract, strongly, the glute of the down leg while also engaging the abdominals. You are trying to slightly rotate your hip backwards (as if 'spilling water' out of the back of your hips). Note the amount of tension, if any, felt in the front of the leg (hip flexors or quadriceps).

3. Repeat with the opposite leg down.

CORRECTIVE ACTIONS
- Provide TSM to asymmetrical areas of tension and re-test.

#9: **Heel to Glute**

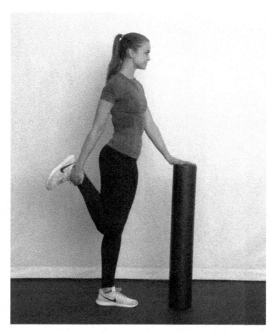

PLIABILITY GOAL
• Symmetry of soft-tissue restrictions

SELF-TEST INSTRUCTIONS
1. While standing with one hand on support, pull one heel towards the glute, holding the ankle. Take note of the tension in the front of the leg, the quadricep or hip flexor.

2. Repeat with the opposite leg.

CORRECTIVE ACTIONS
• Provide TSM to asymmetrical areas of tension and re-test.

RANGE OF MOTION SELF-TESTS

#10: **Toe Reaches**

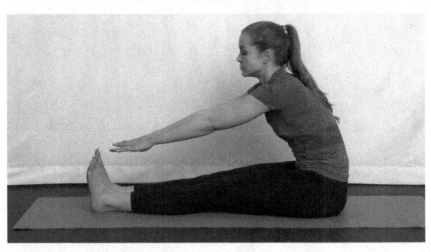

PLIABILITY GOAL
• Symmetry of soft-tissue restrictions

SELF-TEST INSTRUCTIONS
1. With legs together, slowly lean forward, reaching towards your toes.

2. If specific, asymmetrical soft-tissue restriction was felt, perform TSM on the area and retest.

3. With one leg bent, reach both hands towards the foot of the straight leg.

4. Repeat #3 with the opposite leg.

CORRECTIVE ACTIONS
• Provide TSM to asymmetrical areas of tension and re-test.

#11: **Hamstring Active-Isolated Stretch**

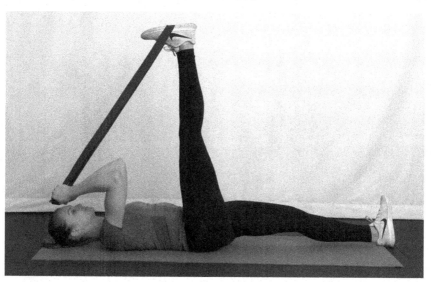

PLIABILITY GOAL

- Symmetry of soft-tissue restrictions

SELF-TEST INSTRUCTIONS

1. While lying down, with a band around one foot, slowly lift the leg while keeping the leg straight at all times (contract quads). Pull the band slightly to increase the stretch.

2. Repeat with the opposite leg.

CORRECTIVE ACTIONS

- Provide TSM to asymmetrical areas of tension and re-test.

#12: **Hip Excursions**

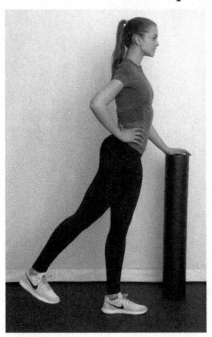 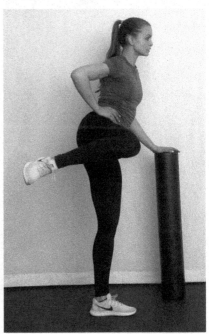

PLIABILITY GOAL

- Symmetry of soft-tissue restrictions

SELF-TEST INSTRUCTIONS

1. While standing on one leg, perform a series of movements of the free leg, comparing with the opposite leg for each:

    - Knee circles forward and backward

    - Straight leg lift up, behind, out to the side

    - Straight leg circles forward and backward

CORRECTIVE ACTIONS

- Provide TSM to asymmetrical areas of tension and re-test.

#13:
Wall-Push Calf Stretch

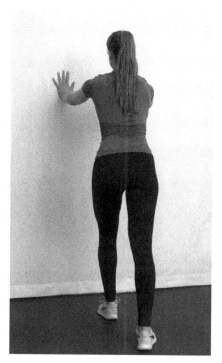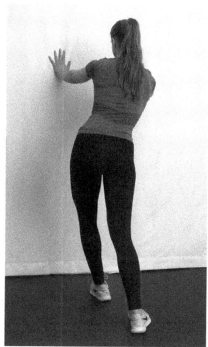

PLIABILITY GOAL
- Symmetry of soft-tissue restrictions

SELF-TEST INSTRUCTIONS
1. With one leg forward and while keeping the back leg straight (engage quads!) slowly move the hips forward toward the wall. Next, move the hips right, and then left. Note where/if tension occurs in the calf of the back leg.
2. Repeat now with the other leg back, noting if that same tension occurs and at the same angle.

CORRECTIVE ACTIONS
- Provide TSM to asymmetrical areas of tension and re-test.

#14: **Shin Walk**

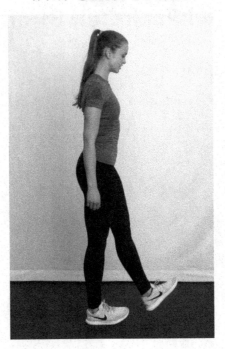

PLIABILITY GOAL
- Symmetry of soft-tissue restrictions

SELF-TEST INSTRUCTIONS
1. Slowly walk on your heels, lifting your toes up as much as possible by contracting your shins (anterior tibialis).

CORRECTIVE ACTIONS
- Provide TSM to asymmetrical areas of tension and re-test.

#15: **Foot/Toe Excursions**

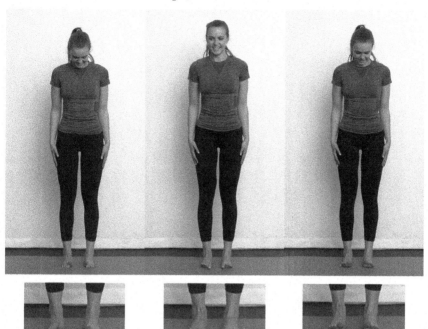

PLIABILITY GOAL
- Symmetry of soft-tissue restrictions

SELF-TEST INSTRUCTIONS
While standing, attempt the following:
1. Lift your big toes up while keeping little toes down. Keep the ball of the foot down and try not to roll your ankle out.
2. Lift little toes up, big toe stays down. Try not to roll your ankles in.
3. Lift all toes up and spread them out as much as possible.
4. Roll your feet out and stand on the outside of your feet. Clench your arches strongly.

CORRECTIVE ACTIONS
- Provide TSM to asymmetrical areas of tension and re-test.

▶ SELF-TESTS:
STRENGTH

For many years, lower body strength training was often avoided by long distance runners. 'Why work the legs with weights when you are running on them every day?' That was the prevailing logic. Today, though, it is clear that times have changed. Advances in science and training theory have shown unequivocally how beneficial strength conditioning is to injury prevention and performance. In fact, it has now become a staple for elite distance runners throughout the world, with many of these elites posting their routines online for runners to learn and implement.

Now, before training for the next Olympics with 205 lbs. deadlifts—something elite marathoners like Jordan Hasay does, and who herself weighs around 100 lbs.—let's move that cart back behind the horse. In this case, we'll call your newly developed strength that can carry you to glory, the cart, and your pliability, the horse. That means pliability leads the charge! Pliability must be in place *before* you start strength training. Otherwise, without optimal circulation, without an inflammation-free system, without a fully functioning and healthy muscle, your gains will be limited no matter how hard you push yourself at the gym.

Adam, 32, runs only for recreation, about three miles two to three days per week. He wants to get faster but does not really want to run much more than he is, so he tries throwing in some strength exercises. He notices some gains at the beginning but they quickly plateau. He is disappointed but wonders if there is something he could do better. It is at this stage that we meet. About halfway through our time together I have him do some simple single leg squats. I ask him to take each leg to the same feeling of fatigue (around 80 percent fatigue). He concentrates on feeling this 80 percent type of fatigue and stops at 12 for the left. With equal concentration he stops at 25 for the right. A major difference in strength, right!? Maybe, but maybe not. I then have him over on the foam roller and sure enough the left quadriceps is significantly less pliable than the right. I talk through the TSM approach and he spends about 2 minutes applying the cycle of 5 seconds compression with 2 seconds rest. He then re-tests the single leg squats on the left leg and immediately he notices he got to 12 much easier, and he eventually stops at 22. So did he really gain strength? Absolutely not. He simply improved muscle coordination, and muscle bioenergetics by improving his pliability!

In *Pliability for Runners,* strength exercises are first treated as another test of pliability, not as a way to get stronger. Gaining strength is important for performance, but it is still only a small percentage when compared to the accumulative effect of consistent aerobic running. Of course, to be consistent with our running we need to be, and stay, healthy. Given this hierarchy, runners should first view strength exercises as an opportunity to catch and fix your soft-tissue imbalances, as most injuries will stem from these. Single leg strength exercises, in particular, can expose more acute areas of tension than a foam roller, as well as different areas than those found from a ROM test. As with the ROM tests, the strength self-tests are using functional movements similar to the act of running to decipher which areas lack pliability and therefore need our attention. Let's go through the first strength self-test together.

#16: **Chest Press**

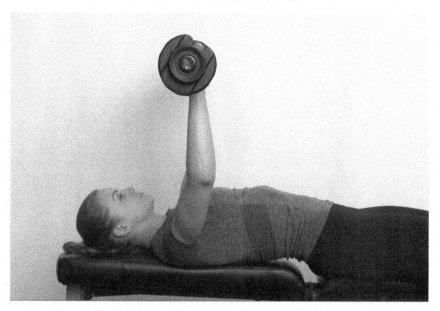

PLIABILITY GOALS

- No tension/restrictions
- Symmetry of location of fatigue

STRENGTH GOAL

- Two sets of 12–15 reps to moderate fatigue with symmetry of strength (right and left arms fatigue at the same rate)

SELF-TEST INSTRUCTIONS

1. While lying and holding dumbbells above you, as shown, slowly lower your arms until dumbbells are chest level—so the elbows drop low and you feel a stretch in the chest.

2. Return your arms to the vertical position and repeat until moderate high fatigue is felt (when you stop you should feel you could still do 3–4 more reps).

CORRECTIVE ACTIONS

- Provide TSM to asymmetrical areas of tension or fatigue.
- Build symmetry of strength through weak-led strengthening.

STRENGTH SELF-TESTS

#16: CHEST PRESS WALKTHROUGH

While lying and holding dumbbells above you, as shown, slowly lower your arms until dumbbells are chest level — so the elbows drop low and you feel a stretch in the chest.

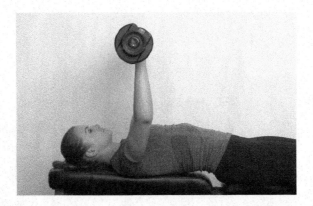

Return your arms to the vertical position and repeat until moderate high fatigue is felt (when you stop you should feel you could still do 3–4 more reps).

While performing the exercise pay close attention to symmetry of movement — arms lower at the same rate, elbows reach the same low point, etc. Were there any tensions that came up on one side more than the other? Perhaps in the shoulder, a pinching in the back, or stretch in the chest? Did one side fatigue in a specific area, where the other side did not fatigue? If so, find a position where that area is loosened and slackened, and apply direct pressure. If there is more than a 2 out of 10 discomfort, and this is more than what the same area on the other side feels like, pliability is our next check.

For example, perhaps there is an uncomfortable pinching in the back of the right shoulder blade when you lower your elbows down. In this case, apply TSM in a position similar to TSM position #9 (page 54, and shown on next page) .

Next, after applying TSM, re-test the Chest Press exercise. Has that tension in the right shoulder improved? If so, continue to perform the self-test and related TSM each day until the movements feel symmetrical.

STRENGTH SELF-TESTS

Wait, I hear you say. Upper body pliability work, really?! The average weight of an arm for a 150 lbs. person is 8 lbs. Imagine if you ran with an 8 lbs. dumbbell taped to the *front* of your right shoulder and another 8 lbs. dumbbell taped to the *back* of your left shoulder. You might end up running in circles! The fact is, many repetitive motion injuries stem from asymmetrical tension in the upper body, shoulders, and arms. Running is a full-body activity against gravity, with every muscle group reacting to each other, therefore the entire body must be addressed, including the upper body!

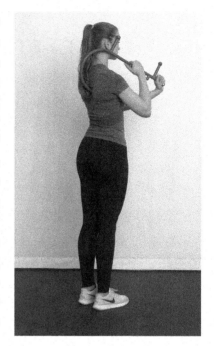

SYMMETRY OF STRENGTH

Not able to find any asymmetrical tensions during the strength self-test? That's great! Now, did you notice if one side simply fatigued earlier than the other? If so, the second, more traditional purpose of strength training, to improve strength, can begin. Given our goal is symmetry of healthy and functional muscles, this should not be through traditional strength training, but through 'weak-led' strength training. Improving asymmetries in strength not only improves our ability to stay injury-free but also improves performance.

STRENGTH SELF-TESTS

WEAK-LED STRENGTH TRAINING

Step 1. Perform the exercise on the weaker side first, taking it to full fatigue. When you stop the exercise the burning/fatigue in the muscle should be moderate high to high.

Step 2. Now perform the exercise on the stronger side, however, the stronger side will only match the number of repetitions or duration that the weaker side could handle.

Step 3. Repeat for 1–2 sets per day and for 2–3 days per week.

Step 4. If the weakness imbalance continues consider the possible adjustments: increase the level of fatigue you take the weak leg to, increase the number of days per week to 4–5 days, or ensure the posture is symmetrically mirrored when doing the exercise.

PUTTING IT ALL TOGETHER

So, in *Pliability for Runners* we are first using strength exercises to learn about more specific areas of the body that lack pliability. After applying TSM and improving the coordination of these exercises, we then test for and improve symmetry of strength through weak-led strength training.

STRENGTH SELF-TESTS: HOW THEY WORK

1. Perform the self-test, which will be a strength exercise you may likely already know. Pay close attention to where fatigue, tension, or discomfort occurs on the right side versus the left.
2. If there is tension that occurs on one side and not on the other, apply TSM to the area, then restart the self-test. Continue this cycle 2–3 times, and once per day, until you feel you are fatiguing in the same areas on each side.
3. Next, perform the self-test again, now taking yourself to a 'memorable' level of fatigue, around 80 percent fatigue. If it is a single leg exercise, perform the self-test on the other leg, taking it to the same feeling of fatigue. If one side fatigues earlier than the other, perform 'weak-led strengthening' until you have reached the goal limit indicated.

BEFORE STARTING ON THE STRENGTH SELF-TESTS, A FEW FINAL TIPS:

- Start right. Ensure your posture is optimally positioned for each leg/side prior to starting the test.

- First movement is critical. Take note of the first micro-second when starting the test, that initial muscle-firing. This moment can be critical as it could be contributing to an altered gait cycle when running.

- Address any unexpected issues ASAP. Compensatory tensions (when you feel tension in an area other than the one that you are focusing on) are common and are equally as important. Be sure to address these early/specific areas of fatigue/tension as you would any other area, provide TSM, then re-test, then repeat.

EQUIPMENT LIST FOR STRENGTH TESTS

2 resistance tubes with handles (medium and heavy)

2–3 resistance loops of varying resistances

Dumbbells that are at least 10 lbs. each

Stair/step at least 4 inches high

KEY FOR STRENGTH SELF-TESTS

TSM = targeted self-massage (pages 51–57)

ROM = range of motion

reps = repetitions

min = minutes

sec = seconds

R = right

L = left

lbs. = pounds

EXERTION LEVEL DEFINITIONS FOR STRENGTH SELF-TESTS

MODERATE. When reaching moderate fatigue you are simply starting to become acutely aware of fatigue. It is starting to clearly set in, but you are still comfortable going forward another 5–10 reps or 5–20 seconds.

MODERATE HIGH. For moderate high you are starting to look to the end, hoping to be done soon. You are definitely fatiguing, and fatiguing quickly. You could, though, push through a couple more reps or 3–5 seconds if needed.

HIGH. Here you have taken yourself very close to your limit. You feel specific muscle burn in the area you are working on.

#17: **Shoulder Press**

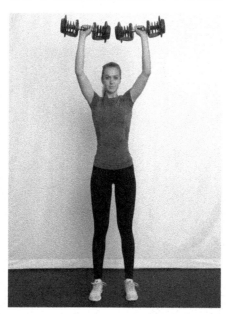

PLIABILITY GOALS

- No tension/restrictions
- Symmetry of location of fatigue

STRENGTH GOAL

- 2 sets of 12–15 reps to moderate fatigue with symmetry of strength (right and left arms fatigue at the same rate)

SELF-TEST INSTRUCTIONS

1. While standing, engage the core so the lower back is braced. Hold two dumbbells at shoulder height.

2. Straighten the arms above your head, as shown.

3. Lower your hands back to shoulder height and repeat until moderate high fatigue is felt (when you stop you should feel you could still do 3–4 more reps).

CORRECTIVE ACTIONS

- Provide TSM to asymmetrical areas of tension or fatigue.
- Build symmetry of strength through weak-led strengthening.

#18: **Reverse Pec Fly**

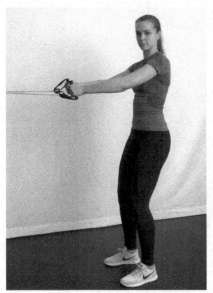 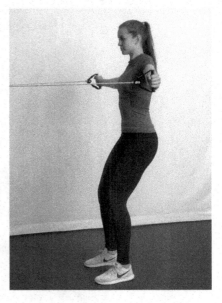

PLIABILITY GOALS

- No tension/restrictions
- Symmetry of location of fatigue

STRENGTH GOAL

- 2 sets of 12–15 reps to moderate fatigue with symmetry of strength

SELF-TEST INSTRUCTIONS

1. When standing as shown, in a quarter squat position with core engaged, hold your arms out straight in front of you while holding a resistance tube.
2. Now, pull your arms back while keeping your arms straight and out wide, away from your body, as much as possible (try NOT to pinch your shoulder blades together).
3. Slowly bring your arms back to in front of you and repeat until moderate high fatigue is felt (when you stop you should feel you could still do 3–4 more reps).

CORRECTIVE ACTIONS

- Provide TSM to asymmetrical areas of tension or fatigue.
- Build symmetry of strength through weak-led strengthening.

#19: **Hip Drives** *(Single Leg Bridge)*

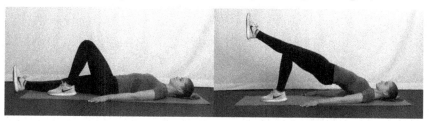

PLIABILITY GOALS

- No tension/restrictions
- Symmetry of location of fatigue

STRENGTH GOAL

- 1 set of 35 reps/leg to moderate high fatigue with symmetry of strength

SELF-TEST INSTRUCTIONS

1. While lying down, as shown, bring the heel of the bent leg close to your body such that if you reach down with a fully extended arm you can just barely touch your heel with your fingertips.

2. Now, with arms out to the side, engage the hamstrings and glutes of the bent leg and drive your hips up towards the ceiling until there is a straight line of the bent leg from the knee to the hip, to the shoulder.

3. Lower and repeat until moderate fatigue.

4. Repeat with other leg.

CORRECTIVE ACTIONS

- Provide TSM to asymmetrical areas of tension or fatigue.
- Build symmetry of strength through weak-led strengthening.

STRENGTH SELF-TESTS

#20: **HAM** *(Hip Abductor Manual)*

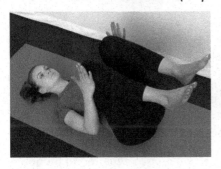 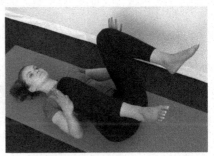

PLIABILITY GOALS

- No tension/restrictions
- Symmetry of location of fatigue

STRENGTH GOAL

- Symmetry of strength with strong manual force in all 3 positions

SELF-TEST INSTRUCTIONS

1. Lie with your knees above chest and fist width apart. Place your forearms next to knees.

2. Press your arms against your legs while pressing your legs against your arms. Nothing should move but there should be strong engagement of your chest, arms, and lateral hip muscles. Hold for 10 seconds or until moderate fatigue.

3. Pay attention to R vs L hip firing throughout

4. Repeat hold when legs are 8–12" apart, and again when 1–2" shy of being as wide as possible.

CORRECTIVE ACTIONS

- Provide TSM to asymmetrical areas of tension or fatigue.
- Build symmetry of strength through weak-led strengthening.

#21: **Clams**

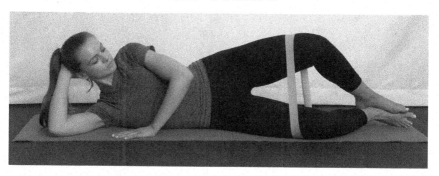

PLIABILITY GOALS

- No tension/restrictions
- Symmetry of location of fatigue

STRENGTH GOAL

- 2 sets of 12–15 reps/leg to moderate fatigue with medium-heavy band, with symmetry of strength

SELF-TEST INSTRUCTIONS

1. While lying on your side, place a resistance loop around your knees with the legs bent.

2. Without rotating your hips/trunk back, lift the top leg up as much as possible.

3. Hold for 1 sec then return to starting position and repeat until moderate fatigue.

4. Repeat with the opposite leg.

CORRECTIVE ACTIONS

- Provide TSM to asymmetrical areas of tension or fatigue.
- Build symmetry of strength through weak-led strengthening.

#22: **AMPL: A** *(Anterior)*

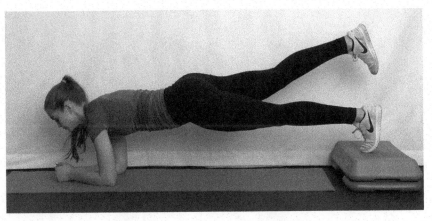

PLIABILITY GOALS

- No tension/restrictions
- Symmetry of location of fatigue

STRENGTH GOAL

- 1 set of a 60 sec hold/leg, with symmetry of strength

SELF-TEST INSTRUCTIONS

1. With your feet on a rise such that your body is parallel to the ground, lift one leg up while keeping the core engaged (back stays flat).
2. Hold this position until moderate high fatigue.
3. Rest for 1 minute, then repeat with the opposite leg down.

CORRECTIVE ACTIONS

- Provide TSM to asymmetrical areas of tension or fatigue.
- Build symmetry of strength through weak-led strengthening.

#23: **Tucked Push**

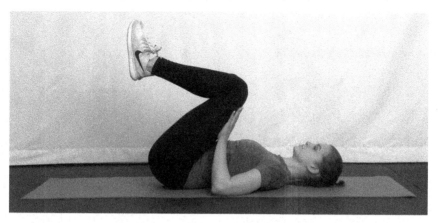

PLIABILITY GOALS
- No tension/restrictions
- Symmetry of location of fatigue

STRENGTH GOAL
- Symmetry of strength with maximum pressure for 10 seconds

SELF-TEST INSTRUCTIONS
1. While lying on your back, bring your knees close to your chest and place your hands on the thighs.
2. Press your hands strongly against the thighs, as if trying to push your legs down, while resisting with your legs (hip flexors engage). Note, this is an isometric hold, so nothing should move.
3. Hold for 5–10 seconds for 3 reps with increasing pressure: light, medium, heavy.

CORRECTIVE ACTIONS
- Provide TSM to asymmetrical areas of tension or fatigue.
- Build symmetry of strength through weak-led strengthening.

STRENGTH SELF-TESTS

#24: **Knee Drives**

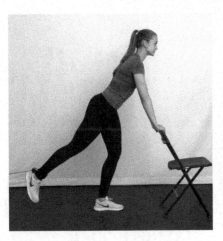 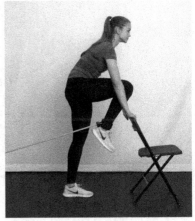

PLIABILITY GOALS

- No tension/restrictions
- Symmetry of location of fatigue

STRENGTH GOAL

- 1 set of 25–30 reps/leg to moderate fatigue with symmetry of strength

SELF-TEST INSTRUCTIONS

1. While standing (as shown) with a resistance tube around one ankle and connected to a support 2–6″ above the ground and behind you, pull the knee up into a running position.

2. Slowly return the leg back to an extended position behind you and repeat. Take 1 sec to lift, 1 sec hold, and 2–3 seconds to lower.

3. Pay close attention to keeping the leg steady (not rotating in or out) at all times.

4. Continue until moderate fatigue.

5. Repeat with the other leg.

CORRECTIVE ACTIONS

- Provide TSM to asymmetrical areas of tension or fatigue.
- Build symmetry of strength through weak-led strengthening.

#25: **Heel Drops**

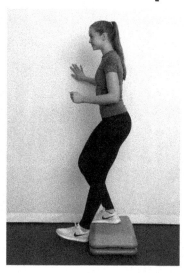

PLIABILITY GOALS

- No tension/restrictions
- Symmetry of location of fatigue

STRENGTH GOAL

- 1 set of 80 reps/leg to moderate fatigue with symmetry of strength

SELF-TEST INSTRUCTIONS

1. While standing on one leg on a stair 4–6″ high, and with the other leg straight and extended in front of you, lower to a position where the knee of the stance leg is 1–2″ in-front of the toes of the same leg, and/or until the heel of the free leg touches the ground.
2. Push back up to a straight position by engaging only the quadriceps (front of the leg) of the stance leg.
3. Repeat until moderate fatigue.
4. Repeat with the other leg.

CORRECTIVE ACTIONS

- Provide TSM to asymmetrical areas of tension or fatigue.
- Build symmetry of strength through weak-led strengthening.

#26: **Single Leg Squats**

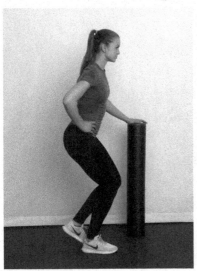
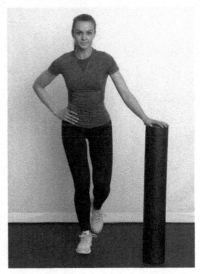

PLIABILITY GOALS
- No tension/restrictions
- Symmetry of location of fatigue

STRENGTH GOAL
- 2 sets of 15 reps/leg to high fatigue with symmetry of strength

SELF-TEST INSTRUCTIONS
1. While standing on one leg, slowly lower to a squat position. Keep weight evenly displaced over the heel and forefoot of the foot, and such that the knee does not move in front of the toes.
2. Push back up to standing by engaging the quadriceps.
3. Repeat until moderate high fatigue. Tempo should be: 4 seconds to lower, 2 second hold, 2 seconds to rise.
4. Repeat with opposite leg.

CORRECTIVE ACTIONS
- Provide TSM to asymmetrical areas of tension or fatigue.
- Build symmetry of strength through weak-led strengthening.

#27: **AMPL: M and P** *(Medial and Posterior)*

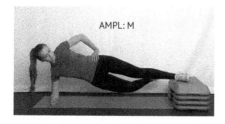
AMPL: M

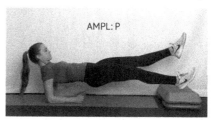
AMPL: P

PLIABILITY GOALS

- No tension/restrictions
- Symmetry of location of fatigue

STRENGTH GOAL

- 1 set of 40 sec hold/leg for AMPL:M, 1 set of 60 sec hold/leg for AMPL:P, with symmetry of strength to moderate high fatigue.

SELF-TEST INSTRUCTIONS

1. AMPL: M—with a step 8–12″ high, lie on your side and place your top leg on the step. Lift your hips off the ground by engaging the groin muscles of the top leg. Hold this position until moderate fatigue, then repeat with the opposite leg.

2. AMPL: P—with a step 4–6″ high, lie on your back, engage your core so back is in a neutral position, place both feet on the step, and lift your hips up by engaging your hamstrings (as if you are pulling your heels down, into the step). Lift one leg up and hold until moderate high fatigue, then repeat with the opposite leg. Note if AMPL: P is too difficult, start with both legs down and build this to 1 min, then start with 2–4 x 5–10 sec holds with single leg. If AMPL: M is too difficult, simulate the exercise while standing with a resistance tube, trying to pull your leg from out to in, against resistance.

CORRECTIVE ACTIONS

- Provide TSM to asymmetrical areas of tension or fatigue.
- Build symmetry of strength through weak-led strengthening.

#28: **Paw Backs**

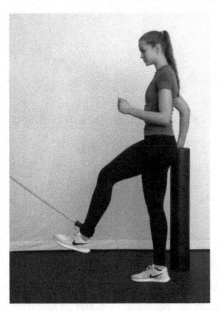 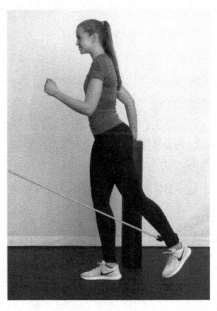

PLIABILITY GOALS
- No tension/restrictions
- Symmetry of location of fatigue

STRENGTH GOAL
- 1 set of 25–30 reps/leg to moderate fatigue with symmetry of strength

SELF-TEST INSTRUCTIONS
1. While standing with one leg extended in front of you, and the resistance tube connected to your ankle and 1–2 feet above ground, pull your leg down and back in a running motion.

2. Slowly return leg back to the start and repeat until moderate fatigue. Tempo should be 2 seconds to pull down, 4 seconds to return to start position.

3. Repeat with the opposite leg.

CORRECTIVE ACTIONS
- Provide TSM to asymmetrical areas of tension or fatigue.
- Build symmetry of strength through weak-led strengthening.

#29: **Ham Curls**

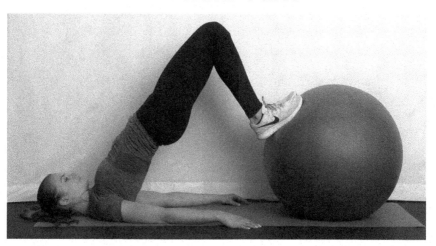

PLIABILITY GOALS
- No tension/restrictions
- Symmetry of location of fatigue

STRENGTH GOAL
- 2 sets of 10 reps/leg to moderate fatigue with symmetry of strength

SELF-TEST INSTRUCTIONS
1. Lie on your back with legs straight and heels resting on a stability ball. Lift your hips up and pull your heels towards your glutes as much as possible. Slowly return to starting position and repeat. Tempo should be 1 second to pull, 2 seconds to return. Repeat for 10 reps.
2. Now repeat the exercise, this time with one leg—opposite leg is raised off the ball at all times. Repeat until moderate fatigue.
3. Repeat with opposite leg.

CORRECTIVE ACTIONS
- Provide TSM to asymmetrical areas of tension or fatigue.
- Build symmetry of strength through weak-led strengthening.
- If single leg is too difficult, first build double leg to 20 reps.

STRENGTH SELF-TESTS

#30: **Reverse Clams**

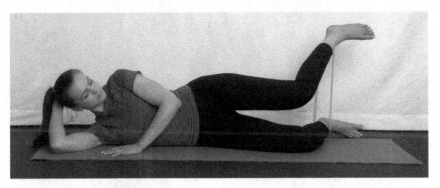

PLIABILITY GOALS

- No tension/restrictions
- Symmetry of location of fatigue

STRENGTH GOAL

- 2 sets of 12–15 reps/leg to moderate fatigue with medium-heavy band, with symmetry of strength

SELF-TEST INSTRUCTIONS

1. While lying as shown with a band wrapped around your ankles, lift the top leg up 2–3 inches.
2. While keeping the thigh of the top leg steady, rotate the thigh inward by lifting the foot of the top leg up. Avoid rotating the hips/trunk.
3. Repeat until moderate fatigue.
4. Repeat with the opposite leg on top.

CORRECTIVE ACTIONS

- Provide TSM to asymmetrical areas of tension or fatigue.
- Build symmetry of strength through weak-led strengthening.

#31: **Hot Salsa**

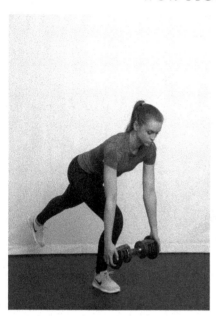 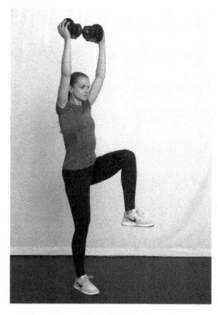

PLIABILITY GOALS

- No tension or restrictions
- Symmetry of location of fatigue

STRENGTH GOAL

- 2 sets of 10 reps per leg with 20 lbs. dumbbell to moderate fatigue with symmetry of strength

SELF-TEST INSTRUCTIONS

1. Step from position 1 to position 2 by engaging the hamstring of the stance leg and keeping the arms straight at all times.

2. Return to position 1 and repeat for 10 reps on the same leg.

3. Repeat with the opposite leg. Note: Start with a 3–5 lbs. dumbbell, then increase gradually over several weeks.

CORRECTIVE ACTIONS

- Provide TSM to asymmetrical areas of tension or fatigue.
- Build symmetry of strength through weak-led strengthening.

STRENGTH SELF-TESTS

#32: **Eccentric Calf Raises**

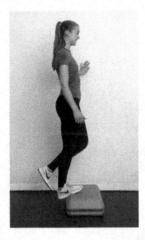

PLIABILITY GOALS
- No tension/restrictions
- Symmetry of location of fatigue

STRENGTH GOAL
- 2 sets of 30 reps/leg to moderate fatigue with symmetry of strength

SELF-TEST INSTRUCTIONS

1. When standing on the edge of a step, stand on one leg (starter leg) and perform a calf raise, holding the top position.

2. Immediately place the free leg (target leg) on the edge of the step in the same tippy-toe position and lift the starter leg off the step. Hold this position for 1 full second.

3. Now, take 5–8 secs to slowly lower the heel of the target leg so the heel is as low as possible, then place the starter leg on the step in the same lowered position.

4. Lift the target leg off so you are now only on the starter leg.

5. Repeat 1–4 until moderate fatigue in the target leg, then switch.

CORRECTIVE ACTIONS
- Provide TSM to asymmetrical areas of tension or fatigue.
- Build symmetry of strength through weak-led strengthening.

#33: **Single Leg Hops**

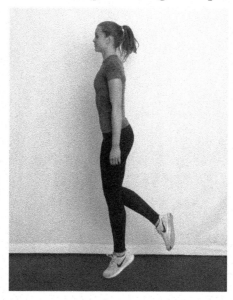

PLIABILITY GOALS
- No tension/restrictions
- Symmetry of location of fatigue

STRENGTH GOAL
- 2 sets of 100 hops/leg to moderate high fatigue with symmetry of strength

SELF-TEST INSTRUCTIONS
1. Hop on one leg, lightly and fast. Foot should only lift approximately ½ –1" off the ground, and at rate of 3/sec (180 hops per minute). Legs should remain straight (quads always engaged) and heel as high as possible (calves fully engaged).
2. Continue until moderate high fatigue.
3. Repeat with the opposite leg.

CORRECTIVE ACTIONS
- Provide TSM to asymmetrical areas of tension or fatigue.
- Build symmetry of strength through weak-led strengthening.
- If single leg hops are too difficult, first build double leg to 200 hops over several weeks.

#34: **Peroneal Isolation Exercise** *(PIE)*

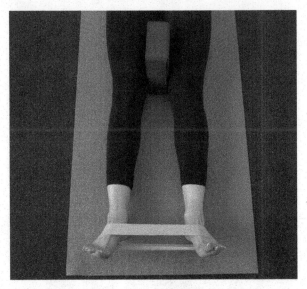

PLIABILITY GOALS
- No tension/restrictions
- Symmetry of location of fatigue

STRENGTH GOAL
- 1 set of 12–15 reps to moderate fatigue with symmetry of strength

SELF-TEST INSTRUCTIONS
1. While sitting as shown, with a block in between your thighs, place a band around your feet when your feet are rolled inwards.
2. Slowly roll your feet outwards, against the resistance of the band, then return back to start. Tempo should be 2 seconds out, 2 second hold in 'out' position, 4 seconds to slowly return.

CORRECTIVE ACTIONS
- Provide TSM to asymmetrical areas of tension or fatigue.
- Build symmetry of strength through weak-led strengthening.

STRENGTH SELF-TESTS

#35: **Shin Lifts**

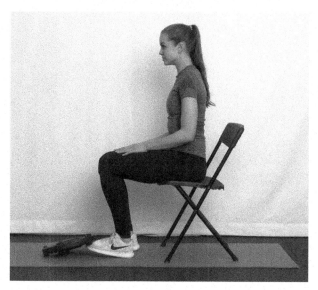

PLIABILITY GOALS

- No tension/restrictions
- Symmetry of location of fatigue

STRENGTH GOAL

- 1 set of 12–15 reps/leg to moderate fatigue with a 45 lbs. weight

SELF-TEST INSTRUCTIONS

1. While seated, place a weight (10–45 lbs.) over one foot. Lift the weight up as high as possible, hold, then slowly lower. Tempo should be 2 seconds to lift, 2 second hold up, 4 seconds to lower, repeat.

2. Repeat the exercise on one leg until moderate fatigue.

3. Repeat with the opposite leg.

CORRECTIVE ACTIONS

- Provide TSM to asymmetrical areas of tension or fatigue.
- Build symmetry of strength through weak-led strengthening.

▶ FINAL CHECKLIST

Y ou have worked diligently to achieve symmetry of pliability, you are strong throughout your body, and you are running injury-free. You have made it! Or have you? For many, it is when you are most fit that you are most vulnerable to injury. After running for several weeks and months you have increased the amount and frequency of force that your cardiovascular system can now endure, which is great! Mechanically, however, any subtle, minor dysfunction that surfaces, and is unattended to, can accumulate to a more severe injury than what you previously may have had. When you are fit your heart is stronger, your cardiovascular and metabolic systems are more efficient, running feels easier and you are doing more and more each week. But are you maintaining responsive tires to go with that new engine?

The next page is perhaps the most important page of *Pliability for Runners*, a checklist of the critical range of motion and strength self-tests that you should be able to test and 'pass' throughout your training. When you are healthy and running regularly, developing the habit of working through this checklist each week can help you avoid the majority of running injuries and allow you to continue to build power and speed.

THE CHECKLIST

RANGE OF MOTION (ROM) SELF-TESTS

Work through each of the following twice per week. These can be split up, e.g. first half on Monday, second half on Tuesday, etc.

1. Standing Torso Twist	page 58
2. Squat Twist	page 67
3. Heel to Glute	page 71
4. Hip Excursions (knee circles forward and backward)	page 74
5. Wall-push Calf Stretch	page 75
6. Active-Isolated Stretch–Hip Flexor	page 70
7. Toe Reaches (legs together, then legs apart)	page 72
8. Supermans	page 65
9. Lying Torso Twist	page 66
10. Knee to Chest	page 68
11. Knee to Chest with Twist	page 69
12. Foot/Toe Excursions	page 77
13. Shin Walk	page 76

STRENGTH SELF-TESTS

Work through each of the following one day per week. These can be split up, e.g. 1–2 exercises per day, or 3–4 exercises for two days per week, etc.

14. Single Leg Hops: 1 set of 60–100 hops/leg	page 103
15. Single Leg Squats: 2 * 6–15 reps @ 4–2–2 tempo/leg	page 96
16. Hot Salsa: 2 * 4–10/leg	page 101
17. AMPL: M and P: 1 * 10–60 second holds/leg/position	page 97
18. Hip Drives: 1 * 10–35 reps/leg	page 89
19. Tucked Push: 3 * 10 sec holds (light-medium-strong)	page 93
20. HAM: 3 * 10 second holds (1*10 sec per position)	page 90
21. Clams: 2 * 6–20 reps/leg	page 91
22. Reverse Clams: 2 * 6–20 reps/leg	page 100

► THE CHECKLIST:
10 MINUTES PER DAY

The Checklist has 22 tests, each comparing right to left, so essentially 44 tests. To cover 44 tests in 10 minutes would take 12.5 seconds per test. Sound unrealistic? If you are making regular improvement, it is absolutely possible! Let's take a closer look at how to approach The Checklist.

First, note the ROM self-tests only need to be done twice per week, assuming that all tests are feeling symmetrical. This assumption stems from the hope that you have already worked daily, and perhaps for many weeks, on the ROM self-test pages to correct your imbalances. If this is the case, the self-tests on The Checklist now serve as a quick 'check-in' to ensure your previously attained gains are holding. If this is the case each test should be very quick, 3–10 seconds each, as you notice everything feels equal and there is nothing to work on.

If something does come up, say after a high intensity run, and now you feel one side is tighter than the other with one of the self-tests, it is time to veer off from The Checklist and address the issue fully. Performing this 'failed' test, and applying TSM to correct the test, now become your daily task until resolved. When resolved, you then continue with The Checklist, picking up where you had left off.

A similar approach can be taken with the Strength self-tests that are on The Checklist. Note these can be done just one day per week, assuming there is symmetry of fatigue and you are able to reach the end-goal limits indicated. If either is not true, move the asymmetrical or weak test(s) to a more frequent habit, now foregoing The Checklist. Through TSM and weak-led training you then work to get the test back to symmetry and to full strength. At this point you can return back to The Checklist and the rhythm of working through these self-tests once per week.

Here is an example:

THE CHECKLIST: SAMPLE WEEK

DAY	SELF-TESTS PERFORMED	TIME
Monday	ROM self-tests (During the 'knee to chest' test, observed that right hip is tighter than the left)	10 min
Tuesday	'Knee to chest' self-test and TSM work	5 min
Wednesday	'Knee to chest' self-test and TSM work	5 min
Thursday	'Knee to chest' work and first four exercises of Strength self-tests	15 min
Friday	'Knee to chest' self-test and TSM work	5 min
Saturday	ROM self-tests ('knee to chest' is okay!)	10 min
Sunday	Last five exercises of Strength self-tests	15 min

The next couple pages show a 'notebook' form of The Checklist, but feel free to make your own!

THE CHECKLIST: RANGE OF MOTION (ROM)

SELF-TEST	REFERENCE PHOTO	NOTES
Standing Torso Twist		
Squat Twist		
Heel to Glute		
Hip Excursions (Knee Circles)		
Wall-Push Calf Stretch		

THE CHECKLIST: RANGE OF MOTION (ROM)

SELF-TEST	REFERENCE PHOTO	NOTES
Active-Isolated Stretch Hip Flexor		
Toe Reach (together, then apart)		
Supermans		
Lying Torso Twist		
Knee to Chest		
Knee to Chest with Twist		
Foot/Toe Excursions		
Shin Walk		

THE CHECKLIST: STRENGTH SELF-TESTS

EXERCISE	GOAL	NOTES
Single Leg Hops	2 sets of 100 hops/leg	
Single Leg Squats	2 sets of 15 reps/leg with 4–2–2 tempo	
Hot Salsa	2 sets of 10 reps per leg with 20 lbs. dumbbell	
AMPL: M & P	1 set of 60 sec hold/leg	
Hip Drives	1 set of 35 reps/leg	
Tucked Push	Symmetry of strength with maximum pressure	
HAM	Symmetry of strength with strong manual force	
Clams	2 sets of 12–15 reps/leg with medium-heavy band	
Reverse Clams	2 sets of 12–15 reps/leg with medium-heavy band	

10-WEEK PROGRAMS FOR RETURNING TO RUNNING

With our daily 10 minute work on The Checklist in place, the final step is to progress gradually with our running such that we are providing a sufficient stimulus and a sufficient recovery. The stimulus is a constant but slight increase in running volume that focuses almost exclusively on easy running over 10 weeks. The recovery involves the off days, the days you are running shorter than you might feel you can manage, and the time spent with The Checklist.

There are three 10-week programs provided: one for the beginner, one for intermediate athletes, and one for advanced endurance runners. It is very likely your ideal program is not listed but is instead a customization of these programs. Adjust as necessary, and trust your instincts. If you find you are repeatedly getting injured, design a more conservative, longer build-up of easy running before shooting for your personal bests.

Note: The strength checklist is shown on the following programs as 1 day per week. As discussed, the self-tests can be split up over 2–3 days as needed, for those short on time. It is recommended to do strength self-tests after a run and with an off-day or light day following.

10-WEEK BUILD-UP: BEGINNER

PREREQUISITES

- Symmetry of range of motion, coordination, and strength with all self-tests listed on The Checklist

- Able to run two minutes continuous pain-free

- Able to dedicate at least 30 minutes twice per week, or 10 minutes per day, to monitor and correct imbalances that may come up when working through The Checklist

This is a program for those who have never run before, or for many years. There is at least 1 day off in between all runs in order for the body to adapt and recover, and to allow time for working through The Checklist. For those with a history of chronic injury it is recommended to re-test any previous imbalances just prior to every run, taking the strength self-tests to a light to moderate fatigue only.

KEY: E = *easy running*   **STR** = *strength checklist*
W = *walking*   **'3*(4W, 1E)'** = *15 minutes alternating 4 minutes of*
ROM = *ROM checklist*   *walking with 1 min of easy running*

10-WEEK BUILD-UP: BEGINNER

MON	TUES	WED	THURS	FRI	SAT	SUN
3*(4W, 1E)	ROM	4*(4W,1E)	Strength	ROM	5*(4W,1E)	
ROM	6*(4W,1E)	Strength	ROM	2*(3W,2E)		3*(3W,2E)
ROM	Strength	3*(3W,2E)	ROM	4*(3W,2E)		ROM
5*(3W,2E)	ROM	6*(3W,2E)	Strength	ROM	2*(2W,3E)	
3*(2W,3E)	Strength	ROM	4*(2W,3E)	ROM	4*(2W,3E)	
ROM	5*(2W,3E)	ROM	6*(2W,3E)	Strength		2*(1W,4E)
ROM	3*(1W,4E)	Strength		4*(1W,4E)	ROM	5*(1W,4E)
	ROM	6*(1W,4E)	Strength		8E	ROM
10E + STR		3*(1W,5E)	ROM	12E	ROM	14E
ROM	3*(1W,6E)		16E + STR		ROM	20E

10-WEEK BUILD-UP: INTERMEDIATE

PREREQUISITES

- Symmetry of range of motion, coordination, and strength with all self-tests listed on The Checklist
- Able to run five minutes continuous pain-free
- Has run at least 80 minutes continuous within last three years
- Has same body weight (within 10 lbs.) as last 60 min run
- Able to dedicate at least 30 minutes twice per week, or 10 minutes per day, on The Checklist

This is a program for those who have run consistently in their past (at least 4 runs per week, for at least 6 weeks in a row). For those feeling 'in-between' the beginner and intermediate plans, consider taking Thursdays and/or Tuesdays off with many of the weeks below. Be sure to adjust the program to how your body is reacting, with the weekly goal being to feel symmetry with The Checklist and ready for the longer effort on Sundays.

KEY:		
ROM = ROM checklist	**W** = walking	
STR = strength checklist	**'2*(2W, 3E)'** = 10 minutes total alternating 2 min walk	
E = easy running	with 3 min easy running	

10-WEEK BUILD-UP: INTERMEDIATE						
MON	**TUES**	**WED**	**THURS**	**FRI**	**SAT**	**SUN**
2*(2W, 3E)	ROM	3*(2W, 4E)		10E + STR	ROM	15E
ROM	20E	STR		15E	ROM	20E
	10E + ROM	15E	20E + STR		20E	ROM
25E	ROM	15E	20E	25E+ STR	ROM	30E
ROM	20E	20E + STR	10E	30E	ROM	40E
STR	ROM	15E	30E	30E	ROM	50E
ROM	25E		40E	STR	ROM	60E
	ROM	30E	40E	50E + STR	ROM	60E
	30E + ROM	40E	30E	50E + STR	ROM	70E
	ROM	50E	30E	50E + STR	ROM	80E

10-WEEK BUILD-UP: ADVANCED

PREREQUISITES

- Symmetry with The Checklist
- Able to run 10 minutes continuous pain-free
- Has run at least 90 minutes continuous within last year
- Has same body weight (within 10 lbs.) as last 90 min run
- Able to dedicate 30 minutes twice per week, or 10 minutes per day, on The Checklist

This is for those who have been running competitively for at least 4 years continuously (e.g. 6 runs/week for 12 weeks in a row, 45 weeks of 5 runs/week in a year). If this program is for you, week 10 should be something you have already done at some point in your past. For those feeling 'in-between' the intermediate and advanced plans, consider taking 1–2 days off during the week and reducing the length of 1–2 runs per week by 10–20 minutes. Be sure to adjust the program to how your body is reacting, with the weekly goal of feeling symmetry with The Checklist and ready for the longer effort on Sundays.

KEY: **ROM** = ROM checklist **E** = easy running
STR = strength checklist **W** = walking

10-WEEK BUILD-UP: ADVANCED

MON	TUES	WED	THURS	FRI	SAT	SUN
10E	15E	20E + ROM	30E + STR		30E + ROM	40E
ROM	30E	40E + ROM	40E	STR	30E	50E
ROM	35E	45E + STR	30E	50E	ROM	60E
ROM	40E	50E	50E + STR	30E	40E + ROM	70E
ROM	40E	50E	60E + STR	30E	50E + ROM	70E
	30E + ROM	40E	70E	STR	30E + ROM	80E
ROM	40E	60E + STR	50E	60E	ROM	80E
20E	40E + ROM	60E	60E + STR	ROM	30E	90E
ROM	40E	60E	70E + STR	30E	50E + ROM	75E
30E	50E + ROM	60E	60E	60E + STR	30E + ROM	100E

▶ FAQS

Feeling stuck? The following pages list common questions I have come across over the years. The answers provided apply to the most common situations and only serve to generate thought and direct appropriate action. In many cases, particularly when improving pliability is not providing immediate improvement, this action involves seeking individual consult from a medical practitioner.

QUESTION 1: *I feel tight, can't I just stretch?*

Unfortunately, that is not always the right path and the research here is perhaps at the most infant stage of all topics discussed thus far. The effectiveness of stretching depends on the type of stretch, intensity of stretch, duration of stretch, direction of stretch, and there is little consistency of these variables from one study to the next. With most studies, even if most variables line up, the results themselves are inconsistent. For instance, in some cases traditional static stretching may help, where the tension is due to very minor fluid/chemical disruptions, but in others stretching is shown to inhibit performance. The most common solution often lies in the correct order of corrective actions, starting with pliability work. In most cases, increasing pliability will increase flexibility and is most often the safer, more effective way to gain a lasting increase in range of motion.

QUESTION 2: *I have considerably less range of motion on one side vs the other, but I don't feel any soft-tissue tension contributing to this? It is as if I simply cannot move any further, it just stops. What's up with that?*

If there is an imbalance in ROM, without restriction from soft-tissue, a structural imbalance may be at play here. Examples are a hip obliquity, where one hip is higher/rotated differently than the other, a structural leg length difference, and scoliosis. If you suspect you have a structural imbalance, first double check the soft-tissue pliability of the areas above, below and around the area of the body that exhibits the ROM imbalance, as always comparing right to left. If no notable pliability difference is found, you may indeed be up against a genetic structural imbalance, or a structural imbalance where 'surface' soft-tissue is no longer the cause. In certain instances, there are quick fixes that may help, for example a shoe-lift, chiropractic adjustment, or surgery. Often, though, these same fixes do not help and thus the injuries continue. If this sounds like you, validate your suspicions by seeing a qualified health professional. In most cases an x-ray would be enough to decipher if and to what degree a structural imbalance is present.

Regardless of a rigid structural imbalance, we still need to have symmetry of pliability and coordination throughout the body. There are plenty of Olympic level athletes that have such structural asymmetries, and can stay relatively injury-free. This is due to the fact that though their mechanics might be imbalanced, their muscles throughout the body are staying pliable, healthy, with full circulation and minimal inflammation. So, in short, if everything else is going well, in terms of pliability, it may be time to move on from ROM tests and into the strength tests.

QUESTION 3: *I continue to work on Targeted Self-Massage for one particular area, but the tension always comes back. I can get it to lower slightly, but after just a short run it comes back.*

It is possible you are working on an area that is tightening up as a reaction to either the posture with which you are landing, and/or excessive tension/vibration/weakness of a nearby muscle. This is why all areas must be worked on and brought to symmetry simultaneously prior to running — i.e. you can pass all of the self-tests in The Checklist. If all areas are healthy and fully functioning, the posture of your gait may improve; and if not, you will still be able to more efficiently absorb and propel forces despite the less-than-ideal mechanics.

Below are some common muscle pairings, where if one area is stiff/weak it will often cause another to follow along:

Lower back/hip flexor

Lower back/glute

Glute/hip flexor

Glute/medial quadricep

Glute/hamstring

Glute/groin

Quadricep/calf

Quadricep/hamstring

Hamstring/calf

Calf/shin

Calf/foot

Some of these pairings work synergistically, where they assist each other in producing the same type of movement. Others are known as reciprocal inhibitors, where each muscle performs the exact opposite function of the other, and thus the pair works together to keep the area stable. If all synergistic and reciprocal inhibitor pairs are symmetrical in pliability yet still the tension returns, it is time for a professional to take a look.

QUESTION 4: *I have been working on strengthening my imbalance but I am not seeing much improvement, any ideas?*

First, let's double check your posture, throughout your body, when doing the exercise. For example, when doing single leg squats, if you are leaning over the right leg more than the left, this will alter the muscle-firing. Or perhaps one hip is out to the side too much, or even rotated down or up more than the other. A great test for symmetry of hip position is the 'cat/cow positions' in yoga (quick video search of this, or 'anterior vs posterior pelvic tilt', may help here). Try these movements focusing on one leg, one hip at a time. See if you notice a difference in the ease or range of motion right vs. left, perhaps one hip can tilt down more than the other? Is tension or resistance felt asymmetrically? If so, apply the TSM method and retest. If not, develop coordination of this movement through daily practice.

If no noticeable postural imbalances are found, and/or the strength imbalance is still present despite improvement of posture, it is time to get clinical confirmation in regard to structural imbalances, neural inhibition, etc. If after a thorough analysis by a physician (including scans/x-rays to decipher possible structural/bone discrepancies) you receive a 'clean bill of health', your strength imbalance may stem from an imbalanced load that you are applying to the ground when running, and of which the root cause is irreversible through musculoskeletal stimulus. At this point it is possible to continue with training and gradually progress so long as you, (1) continue to monitor and maintain symmetry of pliability and (2) continue your weak-led strengthening in order to keep the strength imbalance from progressing further.

If you are diligently doing your homework and still have unilateral repetitive motion strain/injury, a podiatrist or physical therapist may be able to design a customized orthotic that may help balance the difference in force. There are many risks to adjusting to new orthotics so this is, in my mind, a last resort.

QUESTION 5: *I am able to improve my strength imbalance but it always seems to come back after I run for a bit. What's happening?*

It is likely that your running mechanics are loading your legs asymmetrically. First, you may need to keep up with those strength exercises more regularly. Second, if you have checked pliability throughout the body and everything is feeling equal, it may be time to have someone look at your gait to see if an imbalanced load is indeed happening. If so, and if you have worked diligently through all self-tests, you might be a good candidate for gait retraining. More on this with Question 10.

QUESTION 6: *I don't think I know how to do this stuff? What if I can't sense these differences in tension?*

"Trust your instincts and be patient" is common advice that I give, and may be worth considering. Minor gains can accumulate to noticeable improvements with short, focused bouts of attention every day for 1–3 weeks. If, after carefully reading and applying the steps outlined in *Pliability for Runners*, you find you are still unsure about your skills to self-diagnose, it may be time to seek outside help from an effective physical therapist, massage therapist, physiotherapist, or similar.

QUESTION 7: *I'm improving. I am running now without pain, maybe just an occasional tension or minor sensation, but that's ok right? I feel like it is just in my mind now!*

Sounds like you are almost there, but even these minor sensations are noteworthy. Keep in mind, when you are running you are having endorphins and hormones circulate that may be masking the normal feedback you would be getting. So, if a minor feeling makes its way through those masking agents it could very well be important — particularly if you take yourself to fatigue with speed or distance. With this in mind, during the first couple months of running the act of running should serve as another test of muscle functionality, similar to the strength self-tests. This means if while running you feel an asymmetrical sensation, tightness or 'mis-firing', stop running, apply targeted self-massage for 30–60 seconds and re-test by continuing the run. If the symptoms are no longer present cautiously continue on, but if they have not changed or have returned, it is time to stop, go home and re-work through The Checklist.

QUESTION 8: *I know some very good runners that are not flexible at all, they can't get close to being able to touch their toes. Is flexibility important?*

Here is the hierarchy that *Pliability for Runners* is based on:

- Most important: symmetry of pliability
- Very important: symmetry of flexibility

- Very important: symmetry of coordination
- Very important: symmetry of strength
- Very important: high level of pliability (very relaxed muscles)
- Moderately important: high level of strength
- Moderately important: high level of coordination
- Moderately important: high level of flexibility

In other words, symmetry is most important, and symmetry of pliability tops the list. If the pliability is symmetrical but the runner has very tight hamstrings, or is symmetrically weak, the process of very gradually increasing the running (both volume and speed) can improve these areas to the extent needed and in the most functional way — through running!

RUNNERS WHO ARE VERY FLEXIBLE

If we go to the extreme with flexibility, we may lose the strong ground reaction that is needed to both stay healthy and improve performance. For example, if one does hot yoga every day and can wrap their legs around their head, it is quite possible they do not have the elastic stretch reflex in their mechanics. This means when they are running and they bring their knee forward, the hamstrings are so loose they do not provide the quick, powerful recoil to drive the leg down and back into the ground (compare stretching and releasing a rubber band vs. Play-Doh). Without the appropriate stiffness of the hamstrings we lose power into the ground. With less power we lose stride length. With a shorter stride length we are running slower than our potential. Therefore, some tightness is good, as long as when those muscles are in a relaxed, shortened, and slackened position they are loose and compliant to strong compression.

RUNNERS WHO ARE VERY STRONG

Often times runners who get injured think they got injured because they were not strong enough. They then hit the gym, or start doing certain strengthening exercises for what they read was their 'weak glutes', or some other muscle. Unfortunately, this is often putting the cart before the horse and ends up leaving an underlying pliability imbalance unattended to (as discussed in the Strength Self-test chapter). If we put things in the right order, pliability to range of motion to coordination and finally to strength, we are then building our most functional version of ourselves, with optimal circulation, blood chemistry, and reaction to stimuli.

QUESTION 9: *I am a marathoner. During a marathon, my right hamstring always tightens up during the last four miles and causes me to drastically slow down. What can be done?*

When running long distances, particularly over two hours, any deficit in energy will impact your most vulnerable areas first. Imagine a large sponge that is wet but with certain pockets that are less wet, less saturated than others. Now place that sponge out in 80 degrees of dry heat. The water will evaporate equally throughout the sponge and thus the first areas to be completely dry are those areas that started off with the least amount of water. If you have areas that lack pliability, and thus lack the proper fluid contents for full functionality, those areas will "feel" the energy starvation first. To combat this, first, diligently address your pliability imbalances as discussed in this book, and second, practice improving your fluid and elec-trolyte refueling until you are sure you are taking in all that you can without detrimental effects (upset stomach, bloated feeling, etc.). If you watch elite marathoners race, particularly the top runners at a world major, you'll notice they are refueling every 15 minutes (every 5k). If you are pushing yourself to the same exertion, even if it is 8, 9 or 10:00 minute miles, you too might need to move to 15 minute in-take intervals in order to replenish what you are using and to keep your soft-tissue system 'running smoothly'.

QUESTION 10: *I'm thinking maybe my injuries are caused by my shoes. Could this be possible?*

In most cases shoes are not the cause of an injury, but some shoes may expose musculoskeletal dysfunctions earlier than others. If the injury is asymmetrical and came about after switching shoes, certainly go back to the store to try a different pair, but also use this as an opportunity to learn more about the true cause of the injury. For example, a runner may not have an injury, but is running with one hip rotated slightly anterior relative to the other hip. When running, this position results in that leg now extending back, behind the body, more than the other leg. No ramifications have surfaced from this, but one day the runner decides to try a zero-drop shoe for the first time. Now, with more impact on the forefoot and more stress on the calves, this new environment coincides with the altered range of motion of the rotated hip and suddenly the calf of that leg is strained. So, though a more gradual move towards a flatter shoe might be a worthy endeavor, use this opportunity to learn more about why that hip is rotated and the other is not.

QUESTION 11: *What is gait retraining, and should I consider this?*

Gait retraining involves making conscious adjustments to your running mechanics *while* running. This method is gaining more and more support as the results from clinical trials, case studies, and medical research are raising the confidence of physical therapists, biomechanists, and exercise physiologists. There are many inherited risks and a lot to be learned, however, and thus gait retraining is not an integral part of *Pliability for Runners*. To understand why this is essentially omitted here, let's examine the current environments in which gait retraining is practiced.

CLINICAL GAIT ANALYSIS

In the clinical setting, runners are taught how to adjust their stride based on the feedback of visual, auditory, or even sensory feedback. For example, while running on a treadmill the patient might see a real-time graph on a screen in front of them, plotting their knee rotation. Then, they are instructed to run such that the line being plotted stays below a certain level marked on the screen. In some labs the runner may be instructed to run such that their foot-strikes line-up with an auditory beep, or a sound is emitted if their hip is dropping down too much, for example. With new technology there are new and creative ways to instruct runners how to move nearly every week, it seems. Unfortunately, however, the research is at an infant stage, lacking the amount of data/results to necessitate a holistic change in the habits of runners. In addition, many gait-retraining studies are not considering all of the variables that are daily, real considerations for the average and competitive runner. The following lists the most common concerns I have with the majority of gait retraining studies.

The study is done with participants walking, not running. The difference in the amount of force, and how force is applied and absorbed when walking vs running is far too great to draw conclusions from.

The study is done without concern about performance. For example, many studies confirm that running with an increased stride rate reduces ground reaction forces (GRFs). This reduction in GRF then reduces the stress on the knee and tibia. It follows then that running with an increased stride rate reduces the likelihood of a tibial stress fracture or patellofemoral pain. So, the runners are back at it, now running with shorter and faster steps. Some might get compensatory injuries (normally foot and calves due to the common move to a mid- or fore-foot landing) but many runners are indeed able to run more/longer and stay more injury-free. But what happens if these runners want to improve their running? They want to shoot for their PR! In comes the faster running, the longer steps, the greater forces, and unfortunately for many, another injury. The common problem in these cases is that a more chronic, critical postural imbalance was not addressed. Though the stride rate was increased, the runner is still running with one hip dropping five degrees more than the other, for example.

The study is done examining how only certain areas of the body are responding to the altered mechanics. This exposes the runner to risks of compensatory adjustments and injury with more long-term use.

With these considerations it becomes clear the industry still needs substantially more time and money to effectively study gait retraining for runners.

GAIT ANALYSIS THROUGH WEARABLE TECHNOLOGY

Bio-monitoring watches, gyroscope phone apps, insoles, or pants with sensors. These are all out there and being used by runners in an effort to run efficiently and to avoid injury. Runners get notified, while running, with a beep, light indicator, vibration, or voice that their stride is out of balance, the stride rate is too slow, the force is too much on the heel, etc. Then, they may or may not receive some suggestions from the device on how to adjust to correct this. The runner makes the attempt and continues to adjust his or her mechanics until the 'red light turns to green'. In some cases, the runner eventually adopts a new gait that produces only a green light, no beeps, no vibrations. The habit takes hold and the runner is training injury-free, until one day they are not, and an injury has surfaced. Now what? Without having a consistent self-care program in place, where you are continually monitoring your body's reaction to mobility, resistance, and running, you are at the mercy of incomplete science.

For example: That new fancy watch that connects to your feet and speaks to you through your blue-tooth headphones may have been developed based on results of the same lab studies mentioned prior, giving suggestions and protocols that are not taking full consideration of your body, your history, your situation. Perhaps your watch-app shows you are landing on your heel on your left foot, and the right foot points out and makes you run on the mid-foot. So, you rotate the right foot in, or rotate the left foot out, whatever it takes to come to symmetry. But what the app does not know is that your left groin muscle has been chronically tight for the past few weeks due to lower back stiffness that surfaced after doing yard work. You, though, go forward and make the adjustment to land more mid-foot on the left foot, but soon the left groin is not compliant to the change. As a reaction to this you subconsciously engage the left leg external rotators (your glutes, the reciprocal inhibitor to the groin muscles) a bit more. You finish the run with a 'green light', but wake up the next day with a stiff hip, or pain on the bottom of your left foot. You take time off from running, then continue the path of adjusting your mechanics to fit the demands of your phone, following the cycle of adjust, tightness/soreness/injury, rest, adjust, tightness/soreness/injury, rest.

Though the end goal of your digital bio-mechanical advisor might be correct, if all you do is adjust your mechanics to meet this end-goal, the risk is far too great you will be stressing or straining areas of the body that are not used to such a change. You might be over-adjusting, over-engaging, or erroneously altering other components of your mechanics. Given this risk, as well as the current state of research, such wearable technology should not be available to most runners, at any level. The data is either too much for anyone to process real-time while he or she is running, or there is not enough data/feedback to safely react to. However, if you just received a new talking insole for your birthday, ideally you follow these three steps:

1. Learn everything you can about your posture, how you move, your soft-tissue restrictions and imbalances, and your running form.

2. Get confirmation from a trained, experienced health care provider that the correction you are doing is optimal and safe.

3. Commence with the gait retraining while continuing with your twice per week work on The Checklist.

DO YOUR OWN RESEARCH

Some runners might find they fit the description of the subjects who participated in a successful gait-retraining study. Perhaps you exhibit the same gait symptoms, same gait characteristics, and have the same activity level of those in such a study. It then follows that you might expect a similar result. By going forward with the gait retraining, however, it is essentially like taking part in a new clinical trial—where the number of participants is just not enough to make solid conclusions. For some it might work, but for some it does not. For those wanting to give it a try, research nearby hospitals, universities, or physical therapy centers to see if there is a gait retraining component to their treatment protocols, and ask to see the clinical studies behind their proposals.

Gait analysis at the Boston Running Center: Given my above thoughts and reactions to gait analysis, I provide a custom-crafted version of gait analysis at the Boston Running Center. Here the results of the analysis serve mainly as a baseline from which to compare results after the participant has attained symmetry of pliability and strength. I look to answer the questions, 'What is happening, from a static and dynamic postural viewpoint? Why is this happening and is it or will it contribute to injury? How can this be corrected, and should it be?'.

▶ PLIABILITY FOR JUNIOR ATHLETES

A study in 2010 calculated that children ages 8–18 spend an average of 7.5 hours per day in front of a screen — an amount that has very likely gone up since. From 1994 to 2007, a separate study found a 34 percent increase in running-related injuries among 12–14-year-olds. So, we have an increase in screen-time alongside an increase in running injuries. Kids are putting themselves in contorted positions, where they are sedentary, likely leaning over, head tilted back, etc., for longer and longer periods of time. Then some of these kids are putting their contorted bodies into action with sport and running and the injury rates are increasing. Can we safely connect the dots?

Today, perhaps for the first time, monitoring and improving pliability for youth runners is just as important as for adults. Cross-country and track high school runners are getting injured just as often as adults, and the cause is often exactly the same. Kids lack solid home-care habits and combine this with doing 'too much too soon' within their training, like not running enough over the summer then going right into full-on cross-country practice! Take care of even one of these causes and there is a significant reduction in injury-rates.

Some kids may not really be into the idea of self-massage and finding small differences in tension. In fact, in most cases, as with adults, kids do not 'jump on board' the *Pliability for Runners* approach until after they get injured. To help ease into the concepts of this book, and establish a simple, yet effective habit to sustain throughout the competitive season, we'll stick to the basics. The below positions are a great introduction into the idea of monitoring right verses left pliability.

GLUTES

Keep your weight over one glute only to fully assess the tension. Now very slowly rotate your body clockwise, then counterclockwise. Then glide your body right then left along the foam roll. Then, again very slowly, roll forward then backwards on the roll. Switch sides and repeat.

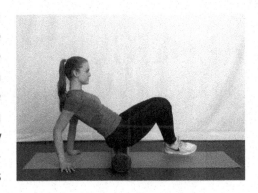

LOWER BACK

Slightly rotate so the pressure is just to the side of the spine on one side. Now slowly roll up and down on the foam roll. Switch sides and repeat.

UPPER BACK

Focus on the areas around rear shoulder and then the back of the armpit. Slowly roll up and down. Switch sides and repeat.

QUADRICEPS

Focus on three areas for each quad. AREA 1: hip flexor (first 2–6″ below the hip bone) AREA 2: mid quad (halfway between hip and knee) AREA 3: lower quad (just above knee)

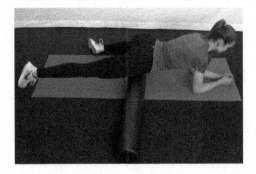

HAMSTRINGS

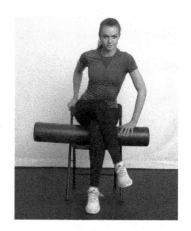

With legs crossed and body weight positioned over one leg, all the pressure should be felt from the foam roller going into your mid-thigh/mid-hamstring area. Now very slowly rotate your body right to left, glide right to left, and/or roll forwards and backwards. Switch sides and repeat.

CALVES

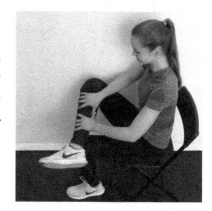

With strong pressure of your hands and thumbs, and while in one or more of the positions shown, assess the tension/pliability throughout the calf.

SHINS

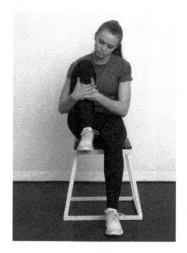

With palm of the opposite hand pressing the fingers of the placed hand, strongly apply pressure and assess the tension/ pliability of the shin.

JUNIOR ATHLETE PLIABILITY CHECKLIST

The below chart is a great habit for junior athletes to work through at least once per week. If anything is unbalanced by more than 1 (refer to the scale on page 39) the more restrictive side should be worked on with TSM (see pages 51–57) daily until symmetrical. For those junior athletes who are well organized, ambitious, and determined to become the fastest runner they can, stick with The Checklist on page 108!

JUNIOR ATHLETE PLIABILITY CHECKLIST

AREA	REFERENCE PHOTO	RIGHT 0–10	LEFT 0–10
Glutes			
Lower Back			
Upper Back			
Quadriceps		upper ____ mid____ lower ____	upper ____ mid____ lower ____

JUNIOR ATHLETE PLIABILITY CHECKLIST

AREA	REFERENCE PHOTO	RIGHT 0-10	LEFT 0-10
Hamstrings			
Calves			
Shins			

▶ PLIABILITY FOR EXPLOSIVE SPORT ATHLETES

Hello soccer, lacrosse, field hockey, football, basketball, hockey, and baseball players. First of all, welcome to this niche book meant for endurance runners. I am curious how you found yourself here. However, I am aware that some runners play other sports (as I myself do) and some explosive sport folks run for aerobic fitness or even get a bit competitive with endurance running. Over the past 16 years I have worked with dozens of ball sport players and have found, as you might guess, similar trends. Asymmetrical hypertensions, a subsequent postural distortion and biomechanical imbalance, and an eventual over-load/injury into one leg. Certainly, the same self-tests and checklist in *Pliability for Runners* can be extremely helpful for these types of athletes — as in nearly all sports the entire body is being used just as it is with endurance running. However, what follows is a more concise, introductory sport-specific checklist that can be used in the same manner as The Checklist. Here is a quick reminder of how and what to do with the ROM and strength self-tests.

ROM SELF-TESTS: EACH MOVEMENT IS FIRST PERFORMED AS A TEST, COMPARING RIGHT TO LEFT FOR SYMMETRY OF RANGE OF MOTION. TSM is applied to restricted areas and the movement is retested. Repeat daily until the test feels symmetrical without applying TSM, then repeat the test 1–2 days per week.

STRENGTH SELF-TESTS: PERFORM EACH EXERCISE NOTING IF FATIGUE OCCURS IN THE SAME AREA OF THE BODY. If a more acute area fatigues on one side, check for pliability by pressing into the area. If there is more tension than on the other side, perform TSM on the restricting area, then repeat the exercise. Repeat daily until the areas of fatigue are symmetrical. If/when the areas of fatigue are symmetrical, take each side to the same level of fatigue (80 percent fatigue). If one side fatigues earlier than the other, begin weak-led training (page 84).

SOCCER PLIABILITY CHECKLIST

AREA	REFERENCE PHOTO	RIGHT 0–10	LEFT 0–10
Squat Twist			
Knee to Chest			
Knee to Chest with Twist			
Heel to Glute			

SOCCER PLIABILITY CHECKLIST

AREA	REFERENCE PHOTO	RIGHT 0–10	LEFT 0–10
SLS			
AMPL: P			
Hops			

FIELD HOCKEY/LACROSSE PLIABILITY CHECKLIST

AREA	REFERENCE PHOTO	RIGHT 0-10	LEFT 0-10
Shoulder Mobility Screen			
Squat Twist			
Knee to Chest			
Heel to Glute			
Shoulder Press			

FIELD HOCKEY/LACROSSE PLIABILITY CHECKLIST

AREA	REFERENCE PHOTO	RIGHT 0-10	LEFT 0-10
SLS			
AMPL: P			
Hops			

FOOTBALL PLIABILITY CHECKLIST

AREA	REFERENCE PHOTO	RIGHT 0–10	LEFT 0–10
Knee to Chest			
Knee to Chest with Twist			
Heel to Glute			
Chest Press			
Reverse Pec Fly			

FOOTBALL PLIABILITY CHECKLIST

AREA	REFERENCE PHOTO	RIGHT 0–10	LEFT 0–10
HAM			
AMPL: P			
Tucked Push			

BASKETBALL PLIABILITY CHECKLIST

AREA	REFERENCE PHOTO	RIGHT 0-10	LEFT 0-10
Squat Twist			
Knee to Chest with twist			
AIS Hip Flexor			
Hip Excursions			
Hip Drives			
Clams			

BASKETBALL PLIABILITY CHECKLIST

AREA	REFERENCE PHOTO	RIGHT 0-10	LEFT 0-10
Single Leg Squats			
Reverse Clams			
Hot Salsa			

BASEBALL PLIABILITY CHECKLIST

AREA	REFERENCE PHOTO	RIGHT 0-10	LEFT 0-10
Shoulder Mobility Screen			
Lying Torso Twist			
AIS Hip Flexor			
Hip Excursions			
Chest Press			

BASEBALL PLIABILITY CHECKLIST

AREA	REFERENCE PHOTO	RIGHT 0-10	LEFT 0-10
Shoulder Press			
Reverse Pec Fly			
HAM			

▶ PLIABILITY FOR JOB-BASED RUNNING REQUIREMENTS

This section is for those who need to achieve a certain running standard as part of a job application, or to perform better at their job. Mostly this includes military and police, but over the years I have come across some unique situations. For example, one person was looking to be more agile so she could better direct her dog in their regular dog racing/agility competitions, and another was looking to improve the way he ran visually so that he was not distracting on TV when he was refereeing basketball games, or another needed to run more as running was the time he used to write his movie screenplays!

Regardless of why you need to run, the most common error I see in job-required running is too much too soon. Typically, I find, this is due to the fact that the person does not enjoy running so will put off the training until the last minute. In these cases, the training starts with too much, accelerates too quickly, and the body immediately starts building inflammation, getting tighter, and fatiguing early. For these folks, I am not about to convince you that running is fun (I even have one of those 'Running Sucks' shirts, and believe and embrace that this is part of the sport). Instead, I strongly urge you to 'attack' your pliability issues multiple times a day. If you are trying to skip corners and 'run less, run faster', keeping up with your pliability, and maintaining symmetry of pliability, might just allow you to get through unscathed.

The following checklist is an abbreviated checklist from page 108. The idea here is that we are emphasizing the most used running-muscles, and checking in on them every day.

MILITARY/JOB-BASED PLIABILITY CHECKLIST

AREA	REFERENCE PHOTO	RIGHT 0–10	LEFT 0–10
Lying Torso Twist			
Knee to Chest			
Knee to Chest with Twist			
Heel to Glute			
Hip Excursions			

MILITARY/JOB-BASED PLIABILITY CHECKLIST

AREA	REFERENCE PHOTO	RIGHT 0-10	LEFT 0-10
Wall Push Calf Stretch			
Shin Walk			
Single Leg Squats			

PLIABILITY FOR MASTER RUNNERS

We all know aging isn't fun. We lose lean muscle mass, our metabolic rate decreases, collagen loss impacts our vision, skin, and muscle function. Running, however, is an activity many can enjoy well into their 70s and some beyond. Yes, speed will gradually decrease (10 percent per decade is a common rule of thumb) but good old simple aerobic easy running is something that we can do throughout our lives. The fact is our body, no matter how old, is always ready and able to adapt to whatever habits we instill upon it. Over the last 30 years studies have unequivocally proven that the elderly who exercise regularly achieve the same 20–30 percent increase in aerobic fitness and strength that younger folks get. So, with this, the main obstacle is staying injury-free and for this we turn back to pliability.

Given the natural loss of lean muscle mass and flexibility, the following checklist emphasizes the lower leg a bit more, as well as the strength self-tests. Also, given the weakening of bones, master runners should be more in-tune with their pliability, symmetrically. That is, if one day both quads feel tight on the foam roll relative to the previous day, that is a clear sign you need to rest, and apply TSM until you are feeling back to your norm.

MASTERS PLIABILITY CHECKLIST

AREA	REFERENCE PHOTO	RIGHT 0–10	LEFT 0–10
Glutes (Foam Roll)			
Quadriceps (Foam Roll)			
Knee to Chest Stretch			
Wall Push Calf Stretch			
Single Leg Squats			
Paw-Backs			

MASTERS PLIABILITY CHECKLIST

AREA	REFERENCE PHOTO	RIGHT 0-10	LEFT 0-10
Clams			
Shin Lifts			
PIE			

▶ FINAL THOUGHTS:
A COACH'S
PERSPECTIVE

For those who may be interested in how I got into coaching, and came to embrace pliability as our fairly reliable savior, the story is not all that exciting. I did not go through some life-altering globe-trotting saga of self-discovery or have a sudden epiphany while watching the sunset over the Pacific. If I did, my story would be at the front of the book instead of way back here! The fact is, the 'ground' I stand on today was built gradually, after many years of learning, listening, practicing, and adapting programs to runners of all ages, levels, and genetics. Below is a brief summary.

After being a competitive runner in high school and college, friends and colleagues caught on to my obsession and asked for tips and advice on how to start or improve their running. Why was I obsessed? For a few reasons, all of which I found are shared by most life-long runners. First, there are many direct parallels between competitive running and life in general. To name a few: the importance of staying disciplined and dedicated to achieving your personal and professional goals, the usefulness of staying relaxed under pressure to improve performance, as well as understanding that failing can provide better feedback than succeeding. Second, the obvious health benefits for the heart, mind, and body. Third, the endless opportunities to unleash my competitive nature, mostly upon myself, and at times with others. Mostly boring stuff, I know, but are all reasons nonetheless that running quickly became, and still is, a given part of my daily life.

Back to my early 20s, and to the questions I was regularly getting from new, aspiring runners. Each of these runners wanted to improve, to run faster or longer. Some succeeded but many referred to an ache or a pain as their biggest obstacle. I recognized their passion for the sport was growing, for reasons similar to my own (more 'boring' people I can relate to!), but they were continually being held up by injury. My concerns and curiosity were piqued. What is it about the sport that I love (and love to hate) that is causing so much difficulty for others?

Over the next few years, I dedicated myself to learning about the variety of reactions to physical stress that occurs from one person to the next. Some folks would excel by following a couch to 5k program online, while others would follow that same program and then get injured. Some could easily handle 40 miles per week, while others would breakdown no matter how cautiously they built up their mileage. I began my very early career as a running coach with one key understanding, or one underlying 'truth' — that the most important factor in reaching one's full potential is staying injury-free. To help keep my runners injury-free, I needed to learn more about them, more about others like them, more about the science of bio-mechanics and more about the applied art of guiding and elevating human performance.

So I set off, pouring through physiology journals, traveling to conferences to learn from the leading minds on bio-mechanics, and most importantly, talking to expert physical therapists, orthopedists, podiatrists, massage therapists, chiropractors and other health care providers who were working with runners. I wanted to know what science has tested and proven in terms of injury prevention, which protocols are successful, and which are not, and why similar cases might have different outcomes.

I began to have more and more runners come to me with chronic injuries in the hope that I could help. Mostly, these runners found me through word-of-mouth — I coached someone they knew who then told them about my focus on injury prevention. I wasn't coaching these runners directly, however, which made things a bit more challenging, but I could at the very least point them in the right direction or to the right health professional. Through hearing their stories, though, I always found that their determination to fix their injuries was extraordinary. Many had gone to multiple doctors, had stuck to their physical therapy regimen for many months, and had also spent loads of money on massage, acupuncture, chiropractor, etc. Orthotics, electrolysis, surgery — they were willing to try anything if it meant it might get them back to pain-free running. However, they were still getting injured. After monitoring and guiding the programs of these runners, I soon arrived at my next 'truth': the only person who can keep a runner injury-free is him or herself. Without the self-administered daily habit of monitoring and addressing emerging and seemingly minor discrepancies in the body, the risk of injury increases dramatically.

As my coaching career progressed, I found myself with two clear goals: first, to do all that I can to help runners prevent injury, and second, to do all that I can to help runners run as fast as possible. I was and still am 'symmetrical' when it comes to these two goals. With a constant eye on both performance and long-term health, I was always asking and challenging my runners with key questions. Did your strength-training at the gym actually improve your capacity to handle fast running? Did those PT exercises actually help you 'engage your glutes'? Did your new theragun actually improve your muscle tension on a permanent basis? Is your stretching routine improving your bio-mechanical imbalance? Given the perpetually expanding universe of easily shared ideas, opinions, and products, holding true to a results-focused perspective became a critical mission of my coaching.

Gradually, over many years (as I mentioned earlier, in this is not-made-for-TV story), my ideas and observations turned into tested best practices. Now, after 12 years of heading the gait analysis lab at the Boston Running Center, I have been fortunate to work with a wide range of runners: from 280-pound beginners who have never worked out before, to the chiseled elite runners in Kenya and Ethiopia, and everyone in between. While working with such diverse people, I learned my next 'truth' — that runners of all levels generally get hurt for similar reasons and that many of these injuries can be avoided with the appropriate self-care skills. Which skills exactly? To learn this, I closely monitored common 'debates' in the industry, such as, is stretching good or bad? Stability or mobility? Press or roll? Massage or strengthen? Pliability or [insert nearly any homecare treatment, exercise, or activity]? The resounding winner of these modality battles was and still is, pliability, with the TSM approach taking the front seat. Though my personal story might not be that exciting, the pliability approach, in my mind, is screaming from the mountain tops in a way that should inspire a movie! Or at the very least, this book.

Today I continue coaching and providing gait analysis through the Boston Running Center in Boston, MA. For more information about BRC and our work, please visit www.bostonrunningcenter.com.

Thank you for reading and thank you to all who made this project possible. Thank you to the runners I have worked with at the Boston Running Center for sharing an interest in learning how to get healthy and stay healthy. Thank you to my long-term colleague and friend Sarah Walker with whom we have navigated through the puzzle of corrective actions for over 14 years. Thank you to the elite coaches, specialists, and world-class runners I have had the privilege to work with and learn from. Thank you to the health care practitioners in the Boston area for having an open mind to collaborate on cases and exchange ideas. Thank you to Bill, Andrea and Dana for the great photos and drawings. I look forward to hearing your stories at pliabilityforrunners.com and seeing you run strong, fit, and healthy for years to come.

▶ REFERENCES

Agresta, C, Ward, CR, Wright, WG, Tucker, CA (2018). The effect of unilateral arm swing motion on lower extremity running mechanics associated with injury risk. *Sports Biomech.* Jun 17(2), 206–215.

Antoniak, AE, Greig, CA (2017). The effect of combined resistance exercise training and vitamin D_3 supplementation on musculoskeletal health and function in older adults: a systematic review and meta-analysis. *BMJ Open.* Jul 20, 7(7).

Ashton-Miller, J. (1999). Response of Muscle and Tendon to Injury and Overuse. National Research Council (US) Steering Committee for the Workshop on Work-Related Musculoskeletal Injuries: The Research Base. National Academies Press.

Behrens, M1, Mau-Moeller, A, Bruhn, S. (2014) Effect of plyometric training on neural and mechanical properties of the knee Extensor muscles. *International Journal of Sports Medicine*, 35(2), 101–19.

Beijamini, F, Pereira, SI, Cini, FA, Louzada, FM. (2014) After being challenged by a video game problem, sleep increases the Chance to solve it. *Plos One*, 9(1).

Benca, E, Listabarth, S, Flock, FKJ, Pablik, E, Fischer, C, Walzer, SM, Dorotka, R, Windhager, R, Ziai, P (2020). Analysis of Running-Related Injuries: The Vienna Study. *J Clin Med.* Feb 6, 9(2), 438.

Bengtsson, V, Yu, JG, Gilenstam, K. (2017) Could the negative effects of static stretching in warm-up be restored by sport Specific exercise? *Journal of Sports Medicine and Physical Fitness*, (4).

Bouffard, NA, Cutroneo KR, Badger, GJ, White, SL, Buttolph, TR, Ehrlich, HP, Stevens-Tuttle, D, Langevin, HM. (2008) Tissue Stretch Decreases Soluble TGF-â1 and Type-1 Procollagen in Mouse Subcutaneous Connective Tissue: Evidence From Ex Vivo And In Vivo Models. *Journal of Cellular Physiology,* 214(2), 389-395.

Boyd, C., Crawford, C., Paat, C. F., Price, A., Xenakis, L., & Zhang, W. (2016). The Impact of Massage Therapy on Function in Pain Populations—A Systematic Review and Meta-Analysis of Randomized Controlled Trials: Part III, Surgical Pain Populations. *Pain Medicine,* 17(9), 1757-1772.

Brown, SR, Feldman, ER, Cross, MR, Helms, ER, Marrier, B, Samozino, P, Morin, JB. (2017) The Potential for a Targeted Strength Training Programme to Decrease Asymmetry and Increase Performance: A Proof-of-Concept in Sprinting. *International Journal of Sports Physiology and Performance,* 24, 1-13.

Carneiro, NH, Ribeiro, AS, Nascimento, MA, Gobbo, LA, Schoenfeld, BJ, Achour Júnior, A, Gobbi, S, Oliveira, AR, Cyrino, ES. Effects of different resistance training frequencies on flexibility in older women. *Clinical Interventions in Aging,* 4(10), 531-8.

Cheatham, S. W., & Kolber, M. J. (2017). Does Self-Myofascial Release With a Foam Roll Change Pressure Pain Threshold of The Ipsilateral Lower Extremity Antagonist and Contralateral Muscle Groups? An Exploratory Study. *Journal of Sport Rehabilitation,* 1-18.

Dalgas, U, Stenager, E, Lund, C, Rasmussen, C, Petersen, T, Sørensen, H, Ingemann-Hansen, T, Overgaard, K. (2013) Neural Drive increases following resistance training in patients with multiple sclerosis. *Journal of Neurology,* 260(7), 1822-32.

Eaton, DK, Kann L, Kinchen, S, Shanklin, S, Flint, K, et al (2012). Youth Risk Behavior Surveillance. Centers for Disease Control and Prevention. June.

Fiatarone, MA, Marks, EC, Ryan, ND, Meredith, CN, Lipsitz, LA, Evans, WJ (1990). High-intensity strength training in nonagenarians. Effects on skeletal muscle. *JAMA.* Jun 13, 263(22),3029-34.

Frontera, WR, Hughes, VA, Fielding, RA, Fiatarone, MA, Evans, WJ, Roubenoff, R (1985). Aging of skeletal muscle: a 12-yr longitudinal study. *J Appl Physiol.* 2000 Apr, 88(4),1321–6.

Halon-Golabek, M, Borkowska, A, Herman-Antosiewicz, A, Antosiewicz, J (2019). Iron Metabolism of the Skeletal Muscle and Neurodegeneration. *Front Neurosci.* Mar 15,13,165.

Hangelbroek, RWJ, Knuiman, P, Tieland, M (2018). Attenuated strength gains during prolonged resistance exercise training in older adults with high inflammatory status. *Exp Gerontol.* Jun, 106, 154–158.

Heath, GW, Hagberg, JM, Ehsani, AA, Holloszy, JO (1981). A physiological comparison of young and older endurance athletes. *J Appl Physiol Respir Environ Exerc Physiol.* Sep, 51(3),634–40.

Heidersheit, BC< Chumanov, ES, Michalski, MP, Wille, CM, Ryan, MB. (2011) Effects of Step Rate Manipulation on Joint Mechanics during Running. Medicine and Science in Sports and Exercise.

Howard, EE, Pasiakos, SM, Blesso, CN, Fussell, MA, Rodriguez, NR (2020). Divergent Roles of Inflammation in Skeletal Muscle Recovery From Injury. *Front Physiol.* Feb 13,11–87.

Kambara, H., Shin, D., & Koike, Y. (2013). A computational model for optimal muscle activity considering muscle Viscoelasticity in wrist movements. *Journal of Neurophysiology,* 109(8), 2145–2160.

Langevin, H. M., Keely, P., Mao, J., Hodge, L. M., Schleip, R., Deng, G., . . . Findley, T. (2016). Connecting (T)issues: How Research in Fascia Biology Can Impact Integrative Oncology. *Cancer Research,* 76(21), 6159–6162.

Larsson, L, Karlsson, J (1978). Isometric and dynamic endurance as a function of age and skeletal muscle characteristics. *Acta Physiol Scand.* Oct,104(2),129–36.

Lenhart, RL, Smith, CR, Vignos, MF, Kaiser, J, Heidershcheit, BC, Thelen, DG. (2015) Influence of step rate and quadriceps Load distribution on patellofemoral cartilage contact pressures during running. *Journal of Biomechanics,* 24, 2871–2878.

Lenhart, RL, Thelen, DG, Willie, CM, Chumanov, ES, Heiderscheit, BC. (2014) Increasing running step rate reduces Patellofemoral joint forces. *Medicins and Science in Sports and Exercise,* 46, 557–564.

Lipina, C, Hundal, HS (2017). Lipid modulation of skeletal muscle mass and function. *J Cachexia Sarcopenia Muscle.* Apr,8(2), 190–201.

Loocke, M. V., Lyons, C., & Simms, C. (2008). Viscoelastic properties of passive skeletal muscle in compression: Stress relaxation behaviour and constitutive modelling. *Journal of Biomechanics,* 41(7), 1555–1566.

Lorenzo, I, Serra-Prat, M, Yébenes, JC (2019). The Role of Water Homeostasis in Muscle Function and Frailty: A Review. *Nutrients.* Aug 9,11(8),1857.

Lu, ZJ (1985). The Yellow Emperor's Internal Classic, an ancient medical canon of traditional Chinese medicine. *J Tradit Chin Med.* Jun, 5(2), 153–4.

Matsuo, Sh, Suzuki, Shi, Iwata, Ma, Banno, Ya, Asai, Yu, Tsuchida, Wa, Inoue, Ta. (2013). Acute Effects of Different Stretching Durations on Passive Torque, Mobility, and Isometric Muscle Force. *Journal of Strength & Conditioning Research,* 27 (12), 3367–3376.

Mau-Moeller, A, Behrens, M, Lindner, T, Bader, R, Bruhn, S. (2013) Age-related changes in neuromuscular function of the Quadriceps muscle in physically active adults. *Journal of Electromyography and Kinesiology,* 23(3), 640–8.

Mehl, AJ, Nelson, NG, McKenzie, LB (2011). Running-related injuries in school-age children and adolescents treated in emergency departments from 1994 through 2007. *Clin Pediatr (Phila).* Feb, 50(2):126–32.

Mitchell, WK, Williams, J, Atherton, P, Larvin, M, Lund, J, Narici, M (2012). Sarcopenia, dynapenia, and the impact of advancing age on human skeletal muscle size and strength; a quantitative review. *Front Physiol.* Jul 11, 3,260.

Morton, SK, Whitehead, JR, Brinkert, RH, Caine, DJ. (2011) Resistance training vs. static stretching: effects on flexibility and Strength. *Journal of Strength and Conditioning Research,* 25(12), 3391–8.

Mount, Fr, Whitmore, MI, Stealey, Sh. (2003) Evaluation of Neutral Body Posture on Shuttle Mission, NASA.

Nelson, N. L. (2015). Massage therapy: understanding the mechanisms of action on blood pressure. A scoping review. *Journal of The American Society of Hypertension,* 9(10), 785–793.

Opar, DA, Williams, MD, Timmins, RG, Dear, NM, Shield, AJ. (2013) Rate of torque and electromyographic development During anticipated eccentric contraction is lower in previously strained hamstrings. *American Journal of Sports Medicine,* 41(1), 116–25.

Pavlov, VA, Tracey, KJ (2015). Neural circuitry and immunity. *Immunol Res.* Dec, 63(1–3):38–57.

Ploeger, HE, Takken, T, de Greef, MH, Timmons, BW (2009). The effects of acute and chronic exercise on inflammatory markers in children and adults with a chronic inflammatory disease: a systematic review. *Exerc Immunol Rev.* 15, 6–41.

Rauh, MJ (2014). Summer training factors and risk of musculoskeletal injury among high school cross-country runners. *J Orthop Sports Phys Ther.* Oct, 44(10), 793–804.

Rauh, MJ, Koepsell, TD, Rivara, FP, Margherita, AJ, Rice, SG (2006). Epidemiology of musculoskeletal injuries among high school cross-country runners. *Am J Epidemiol.* Jan 15, 163(2), 151–9.

Rideout, VJ, Foehr, UG., Roberts, DF (2010). Generation M2: Media in the Lives of 8- to 18-Year-Olds. Henry J. Kaiser Family Foundation.

Ryrsø, CK, Thaning, P, Siebenmann, C, Lundby, C, Lange, P, Pedersen, BK, Hellsten, Y, Iepsen, UW (2018). Effect of endurance versus resistance training on local muscle and systemic inflammation and oxidative stress in COPD. *Scand J Med Sci Sports.* Nov,28(11), 2339–2348.

Santos, E, Rhea, MR, Simão, R, Dias, I, de Salles, BF, Novaes, J, Leite, T, Blair, JC, Bunker, DJ. (2010) Influence of moderately Intense strength training on flexibility in sedentary young women. *Journal of Strength and Conditioning Research,* 24(11), 3144–9.

Siparsky, PN, Kirkendall, DT, Garrett, WE (2014). Muscle changes in aging: understanding sarcopenia. *Sports Health.* Jan, 6(1), 36–40.

Taylor, KL, Sheppard, JM, Lee, H, Plummer, N. (2009) Negative effect of static stretching restored when combined with a sport Specific warm-up component. *Journal of Science Medicine and Sport,* 12(6), 657–61.

Tenforde, AS, Sayres, LC, McCurdy, ML, Collado, H, Sainani, KL, Fredericson, M (2011). Overuse injuries in high school runners: lifetime prevalence and prevention strategies. *PMR. Feb,* 3(2),125–31.

Toume, S, Gefen, A, Weihs, D. (2017) Low-level stretching accelerates cell migration into a gap. *International Wound Journal,* 14(4), 698–703.

Trivers, R, Fink, B, Russell, M, McCarty, K, James, B, Palestis, BG. (2014) Lower body symmetry and running performance in Elite Jamaican track and field athletes. *Plos One,* 17, 9(11).

Wamontree, P., Kanchanakhan, N., Eungpinichpong, W., & Jeensawek, A. (2015). Effects of traditional Thai self-massage using a Wilai massage stick versus ibuprofen in patients with upper back pain associated with myofascial trigger points: a Randomized controlled trial. *Journal of Physical Therapy Science,* 27(11), 3493–3497.

Waters-Banker, C., Dupont-Versteegden, E. E., Kitzman, P. H., & Butterfield, T. A. (2014). Investigating the Mechanisms of Massage Efficacy: The Role of Mechanical Immunomodulation. *Journal of Athletic Training,* 49(2), 266–273.

Wikstrom, E. A., Song, K., Lea, A., & Brown, N. (2017). Comparative Effectiveness of Plantar-Massage Techniques on Postural Control in Those With Chronic Ankle Instability. *Journal of Athletic Training.*

Wilson, JPD, Ratcliff, OM, Meardon, SA, Willy, RW. (2015) Influence of step length and landing pattern on patellofemoral joint Kinetics during running. Scandinavian *Journal of Medicine and Science in Sports.*

Zifchock, RA, Davis, I, Higginson, J, McCaw, S, Royer, T (2008). Side-to-side differences in overuse running injury susceptibility: a retrospective study. *Hum Mov Sci.* Dec 27(6), 888–902.

Zhang, X., Hu, M., Lou, Z., & Liao, B. (2017). Effects of strength and neuromuscular training on functional performance in Athletes after partial medial meniscectomy. *Journal of Exercise Rehabilitation,* 13(1), 110–116.

► ABOUT THE AUTHOR

Joseph McConkey, MS, is a running coach and exercise physiologist, specializing in deducing and correcting causative factors to repetitive motion injury. He has worked with the full spectrum of running athletes, from first-time runners to marathoners around the world, 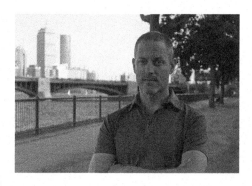 to Olympic athletes at the elite high altitude training camps of Ethiopia and Kenya. He has coached at the club, college, and pro levels and has been the director of the Boston Running Center's Gait Analysis Lab for over a decade. Joseph's expertise on injury-prevention has him regularly presenting at hospitals, rehab centers, running camps, and club events. Joseph holds the highest accreditation by the USA Track and Field Association and the IAAF (the international governing body of track and field), as well as a Masters in Exercises Science with a focus on Injury Prevention and Sports Performance.